PERSONALISED HEALTH MANAGEMENT SYSTEMS

Studies in Health Technology and Informatics

This book series was started in 1990 to promote research conducted under the auspices of the EC programmes' Advanced Informatics in Medicine (AIM) and Biomedical and Health Research (BHR) bioengineering branch. A driving aspect of international health informatics is that telecommunication technology, rehabilitative technology, intelligent home technology and many other components are moving together and form one integrated world of information and communication media. The complete series has been accepted in Medline. Volumes from 2005 onwards are available online.

Series Editors:
Dr. J.P. Christensen, Prof. G. de Moor, Prof. A. Famili, Prof. A. Hasman, Prof. L. Hunter, Dr. I. Iakovidis, Dr. Z. Kolitsi, Mr. O. Le Dour, Dr. A. Lymberis, Prof. P.F. Niederer, Prof. A. Pedotti, Prof. O. Rienhoff, Prof. F.H. Roger France, Dr. N. Rossing, Prof. N. Saranummi, Dr. E.R. Siegel, Dr. P. Wilson, Prof. E.J.S. Hovenga, Prof. M.A. Musen and Prof. J. Mantas

Volume 117

Recently published in this series

ISSN 0926-9630

Personalised Health Management Systems

Systems

The Integration of Innovative Sensing, Textile, Information and Communication Technologies

Edited by

Chris D. Nugent
University of Ulster, Northern Ireland

Paul J. McCullagh
University of Ulster, Northern Ireland

Eric T. McAdams
University of Ulster, Northern Ireland

and

Andreas Lymberis
European Commission, Information Society & Media Directorate-General

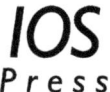

Press

Amsterdam • Berlin • Oxford • Tokyo • Washington, DC

ISBN 978-1-58603-565-5
Library of Congress Control Number: 2005935643

Publisher
IOS Press
Nieuwe Hemweg 6B
1013 BG Amsterdam
Netherlands
fax: +31 20 687 0019
e-mail: order@iospress.nl

Distributor in the UK and Ireland
IOS Press/Lavis Marketing
73 Lime Walk
Headington
Oxford OX3 7AD
England
fax: +44 1865 750079

Distributor in the USA and Canada
IOS Press, Inc.
4502 Rachael Manor Drive
Fairfax, VA 22032
USA
fax: +1 703 323 3668
e-mail: iosbooks@iospress.com

Personalised Health Management Systems
C.D. Nugent et al. (Eds.)
IOS Press, 2005

v

Preface

The International Workshop on "Personalised Health: The Integration of Innovative Sensing, Textiles, Information & Communication Technologies" organised in collaboration with the European Commission, took place in Belfast, Northern Ireland, 13–15th December 2004. At this unique event, addressing personalised health management systems, the workshop endeavoured to promote the synergies between research efforts in three diverse areas; sensor technologies, advanced textiles and nanotechnology and computing. This event followed the International Workshop on "New Generation of Wearable Systems for eHealth" held in Lucca, Italy 2003 and aimed to consolidate the recommendations from this with recent state-of-the-art findings in the evolving health care and health delivery sector, in Europe and world-wide. In addition, the event was timed to coincide with the 4th call for proposals by the IST programme in the 6th Framework Programme of the European Commission. The main goal of the workshop was to facilitate a forum to disseminate progress within the research area of personalised health management systems and to foster collaborations and information exchanges for future efforts. In conjunction with this, the workshop aimed to bring together researchers from academia, industry and clinical health care provision and emphasise the need for multi-disciplinary collaborations in the future developments of personalised health management systems.

The development and advancement of personalised health management systems requires the consideration of advances in sensor technologies and advanced textiles in addition to nanotechnologies and evolving information and communication technologies. We are now living in an environment where changes in healthcare structures and requests from patients to have an increased participation in their own health care are demanding the availability of affordable and readily available personalised health management systems. Recent research has taken us a step closer in providing such solutions, however, efforts are still required to address the issues of integration of new technologies into existing health care practices, implications of interoperability of services, analysis of results following large scale clinical evaluations and development of technology which is small, reliable and affordable by its users.

The workshop programme was designed to facilitate presentations being delivered by leading researchers describing current trends in personalised health management systems in addition to the challenges which are ahead. Areas addressed were Wearable Sensing, Smart Textiles, Standards & Interoperability and Community Health. This book is based on the presentations delivered at the workshop and includes full papers describing the developments and trends in the aforementioned topics. Consideration of the vision of these contributions has provided indications of strategic developments which should be considered to allow the deployment of personalised health management systems into our every day lives.

The Editors
Dr Chris Nugent
Dr Paul McCullagh
Dr Eric McAdams
Dr Andreas Lymberis

Acknowledgments

The editors wish to thank all of the authors for their contributions to this book. In addition, the editors are grateful to Steven Devlin for his continual support in the editing of the papers. Special thanks must also be given to all of the sponsors of the workshop: University of Ulster, Invest Northern Ireland, InterTradeIreland, Department of Trade and Industry (UK), VivoMetrics, Sensor Technology & Devices Ltd., Philips Research Medical Division, BioMedIreland, BioBusiness Northern Ireland, Nanotec Northern Ireland and R&D Office Northern Ireland.

Contents

V. Community Health 2

Personalised Health Management Systems
C.D. Nugent et al. (Eds.)
IOS Press, 2005

Smart Personalised Health Systems: From Gadgets To Better Health

Andreas LYMBERIS

European Commission, Information Society and Media Directorate-General[1], Avenue de Beaulieu, 1160 Brussels, Belgium

The Changing Face of Healthcare Delivery

The healthcare sector has traditionally striven to be at the forefront of most technologies, always willing to try new procedures and spend time and money on medical research like new pharmaceuticals and surgical advances to the benefit of humankind. Yet when it comes to information technology, healthcare has been slow to meet new challenges. To many organisations, IT was regarded as an administrative burden rather than a strategic aid. At a time when governments are faced with ageing populations, future healthcare spending can come only under greater pressures. Thus administrations are faced with the double challenge of improving the quality and accessibility while containing overall costs.

These challenges will be impossible to meet without the deployment and widespread use of fully integrated, interoperable and modernised health systems. This implies fundamental changes in organisation and culture/behaviour and requires significant technological innovation. For example, provision of patient-centric services and faith in technology are critical issues; the full benefits of the information revolution will only be realised when citizens demand that their healthcare providers use the most modern and effective means of delivering services. Another major undergoing shift paradigm is "seamless care", where healthcare professionals have access to all relevant information needed to provide efficient advice and treatment, and where patients and the public have trustworthy information source to assist them in looking after their health.

With the rapid development of the Information society (internet, networking, mobile communications, friendly user-interfaces, etc) during the last 15-20 years, new possibilities are offered for supporting disease prevention and early detection, disease management, rehabilitation and healthy lifestyle. The concept of "continuity of care" is being increasingly adopted by the health community, and in many cases this is best achieved through home-based services, which can be more comfortable and convenient for patient and less costly for health providers. The new means for healthcare and health provision "anywhere, anytime" also assigns new responsibilities for the medical device manufacturer, the health practitioner as well as the patient and citizen. Given the

---

[1] The views developed in this paper are that of the author and do not reflect necessarily the position of the European Commission

decentralised instrumentation (at home, anywhere), the responsibilities of each involved actor become less clear. Personal telemedicine (and eHealth) applications have to comply with user authentication restrictions as well as with personal data protection laws and regulation. Standardisation and certification procedures as well as risk analysis become also crucial. To ensure first class services, the concept of Total Quality Management associated to the traceability has to be applied in all levels.

Information Technologies, Nanotechnologies, Miniaturisation and Integration: the Driving Forces

Healthcare and health delivery greatly benefit from the remarkable progress in sciences and technologies e.g. Information and Communication Technologies (ICT) Micro-Nanotechnology (MNT), molecular medicine, genomics/proteomics, materials science and engineering, and human computer interface.

In today's post genomic era, new diagnostic tools making use of the wealth of genetic data are being developed. All aim to diagnose or detect a disease in its early stage. Different fields in molecular diagnosis lead to the complementary knowledge essential for a complete picture of a disease status. The picture consists of information at genome, protein and cellular levels, unsurprisingly the areas of which new molecular diagnosis focus.

MNT and the integration of MNT-based components in "small and smart systems", in different materials and in large areas (e.g. textile/clothing) enable the creation of enhanced or totally new products for health and healthcare services (and other application domains), ranging from bio-microsystems, biosensors, smart textiles, micro/nano robots, as well as the integration of these sub-systems and devices into the macro world and the body. Applying multi-disciplinarity and system research using a mixture of different technologies and involving users with technology suppliers is a key to realise these integrated systems. Build-in intelligence and clever interfacing of these systems with their environment and with the users is an essential characteristic of their behaviour. Smaller, increased performance, more reliable, lower cost, more portable-wearable, networked, intelligent and emotional products and interfaces are an essential element to implement a user friendly 'ambient intelligent' landscape. These products do and will further change the economic, social and well being context we live in and will generate significant business activities.

Micro-nanotechnologies are at the forefront of current research in the area of in vitro & in vivo diagnostics, point of care biosensor-based systems, wearable and implantable diagnostic and treatment smart systems. They drive interdisciplinary and highly promising developments by researching at the intersection of electronics, chemistry and biology, by pushing the limits of materials and production processes and realising major shift paradigms e.g. from MEMS to BioMEMS and from silicon to plastic. Completely new possibilities are offered in handling biological samples (micro-nano fluidics), in packaging and integrating heterogeneous technologies and systems, in developing micro-nano fabrication techniques for biosensors, in enhancing biocompatibility, in interfacing between electronics and biomedical systems, as well as developing DNA and protein arrays and drug delivery systems.

The large spectrum of systems and applications resulting from the combination of ICT, MNT, biology and healthcare constitute today the so called "personalised smart

Health management systems" area. This area contains worldwide recognised R&D topics e.g. smart wearable monitoring and diagnostic systems, implantable disease management systems, biomedical clothing, point of care in-vitro diagnosis, embedded decision support and other related non research issues. This list isn't exhaustive and given the new R&D topics emerging from the interaction/convergence of well established technologies, it is very likely that the area will significantly expand in the future with new items.

It has to be noticed, that the historical "raison d'être" of this group activity on personalised smart Health management systems was the promotion and support of Intelligent Biomedical Clothing (IBC), an emerging research interdisciplinary topic. This cluster was initiated in Europe by the European Commission, Information Society Technologies (IST) program, starting with related R&D projects funded under the Framework Programmes 6 (2002-2006) and several FP5 projects dealing with home telecare and ambulatory health systems and applications. Other national research projects and stakeholders joined this community building progressively common understanding and clearer vision of the targets and the challenges to be addressed.

Textile, biosensors and Implants: Promising Platforms for Personalised Health Management

A large amount of research and development has been devoted the last two decades to the development of biomedical sensors and sensors-based systems. Several solutions are available today such as, perimetric fixing using the body segments and the circular body part (e.g. head, neck, trunk, arm, wrist, leg and ankle) and networked sensors (e.g. Body Area Network). Hat, belt, wrist, shocks, shoes, headband, smart clothes are used as sensing and measurement device.

One of the main objectives of recent and ongoing research in wearable health systems, in Europe and worldwide, is to increase miniaturisation, system functionality and autonomy with embedded decision support, as well as to enhance user-friendliness and multi-parameter monitoring capabilities.

Today, micro & nano technologies make possible the integration of multiple smart functions into textiles without being a burden. The advantages of this integration are obvious: first, about 90% of the skin is (usually) in contact with textile which is the most "natural" interface to body and second, fabrics are flexible and fit well with human body; they are also cheap and disposable. Currently, the technology vision moves from wearable electronics towards smart fabrics and this vision could be split in three steps: Miniaturization (ongoing), Integration such as embedding electronic components on or into textile with full usability (immediate future) and fiber technology (next future).

Great advances are also achieved in biosensors with the application of microstructures in silicon and, even more competitive, in plastics combined with enzymatic monolayers. The market is expected to grow rapidly; for example in USA the average annual rate is 6,6% and is expected to exceed $ 1,82 billion in 2006. These sensors will open up new possibilities of measuring, currently only in vitro, almost all kinds of data of the human body needed by the medical doctors. The market of biochip systems, lab-on-chip-devices, micro arrays, protein arrays and other related technologies are also on rise (the 5 year average growth rate is estimated at 27,3%). A great effort for further investments is motivated by important technical, ethical and market challenges. More miniaturisation, better integration and packaging and improvement of, sensitivity, stability, selectivity, signal to noise ratio and drift, resolution, dynamic range, gain and dynamic error, are among the major technical challenges for biosensors and biochips.

Telematics implants such as cochlear implants, artificial retina, functional electro-stimulation and drug delivery pumps have also achieved the product phase. They are able to repair or replace vital human functions and interact with the environment and other external devices. Significant research effort is currently put on further miniaturisation, power integration, better biocompatibility and communication features.

All the above technological areas are currently addressed though large R&D and validation activities worldwide. In Europe, the European Commission is funding R&D activities in these areas mainly under the IST (Information Society Technologies) program, *Technologies and devices for micro-nano scale integration* (http://www. cordis.lu/ist/so/micro-nano-tech/home.html), *Integration of biomedical data for better health* (http://www.cordis.lu/ist/so/ehealth/home.html) and under the NMP (Nanotech-nologies, Materials and Processes) Program (http://www.cordis.lu/nmp/home.html).

From Gadgets to Real Systems and Applications

Smart personalised health management systems offer new opportunities for unobtrusive physiological monitoring, point of care diagnosis, early event detection and minimally invasive therapy. The time when medical professionals and other users were considering ICT personal health systems as "gadgets" has evolved. Now, prototype systems have been developed and tested and even some products have reached the market. Such examples are, *LifeShirt*^{TM} *(*Vivometrics Inc. Ventura, CA, USA), *VTAM* prototype (Vêtement de Télé-Assistance Médicale, France) and the Georgia Tech *Smart Shirt* or *Wearable Motherboard (Sensatex, USA).* Recently, *WEALTHY,* an EC funded project combined strain fabric sensor based on piezoresistive yearns, and fabric electrodes realised with metal based yarns, to achieve wearable and wireless instrumented garments, comfortable as a "classical" garment, capable of recording physiological signals. Many other developments are on the pipe line, hopefully expected to deliver the first fully integrated and autonomous biomedical cloth by 2010.

Research has also delivered biosensor-based devices at the point of care for some applications e.g. hand-held device with disposable biosensor for diabetes diagnosis.

Implants and prostheses are more user-targeted, expensive devices and require surgical procedure and strict follow-up, therefore are still not very broadly used. They face also particular problems, e.g. biocompatibility and ethical issues. Nevertheless, products like the pacemaker and cochlear implant are successful business cases and have a well established market.

The future? Collaborative and Interdisciplinary Research

Interdisciplinarity is a key issue when *technology* interacts with the human being.

Some examples of the topics included in the biomedical engineering field, as it is structured today by the International Electrical Engineering Association (IEEE)-

Engineering in Medicine and Biology Society (EMBS), provide an additional argument to this statement: e.g. Physiologic System Modelling, Biomedical Imaging and Image Processing, Biomedical Instrumentation and Biosensors, Therapeutic Physics and Rehabilitation Engineering, Neural Engineering, Healthcare Management Information Systems, Clinical Engineering and Computational Biology and Bioinformatics.

A concrete example of inter-disciplinarity and collaborative research is the Intelligent Biomedical Clothing (IBC) area. Truly IBC that can combine the function of sophisticated medical devices with the comfort and user-friendliness of apparel products could only be conceived through a combination of recent advantages in fields as diverse as polymer and fibre research, advanced material processing, microelectronics, sensors, nanotechnologies, telecommunication, informatics and health knowledge.

The convergence among ICT, nanotechnology, biology and cognitive sciences holds bold promises for the future of our societies, for addressing, through radically new approaches to health and well-being, a number of problems which cannot be solved with existing technologies and methods A collaborative effort in this emerging domain will also reinforce the strength of the related industries in these domains and is a fertile ground for the development of new industries.

Finally, there is need to find new collaborative approaches to facilitate multidisciplinary research, through establishment of physical infrastructures and centres for bringing researchers together and through proper design and set up of end-to-end demonstrators that will prove the concepts and stimulate further research and development.

A Dedicated International Promotion Event for "Smart Personalised Health Management Systems"

International dissemination and promotion events, where all the major actors participate, play a key role for identifying common interest issues, facilitating synergies and collaborations and should accompany any R&D activity in a given area. The first International workshop on *New Generation of Wearable Systems for eHealth* that took place in Lucca, Italy in December 2003 is a significant milestone in the dissemination and promotion of this multidisciplinary area in Europe and world-wide. The follow-up, with the 2nd International Workshop on *Personalised Health through Integration of Innovative Sensing, Textile and ICT*", December, Belfast, Northern Ireland, was of the most successful. It consolidated the great interest of the major international stakeholders for common understanding of the R&D progress and remaining challenges and confirmed the diversity of technologies, disciplines, sectors and actors involved in R&D, promotion, manufacturing, validation, services as well as economic legal and ethical issues. The final goal of this promotion activity is to establish a yearly self-sustainable international event that would allow all relevant actors to discuss and progress research and other support activities at European and International level on personalised health and emerging technologies.

I. Wearable Sensing

Personalised Health Management Systems
C.D. Nugent et al. (Eds.)
IOS Press, 2005

Wearable Healthcare Systems, New Frontiers of e-Textile

Rita PARADISO, Carine BELLOC, Giannicola LORIGA, Nicola TACCINI
Milior-Smartex
Via Giuntini 13 L , Navacchio(PI) Italy

Abstract. There is a growing need of renovation in our health care managing systems; people need to be more interactive and more conscious of their own health condition in a way to adjust incorrect lifestyles, to obtain a personalized therapy tuned to their own physiological reactions and on their own environmental condition. To gain knowledge of a citizen's health status and to monitor without harassing them (until they refuse any medical supervision), a comfortable remote monitoring of important physiological parameters is necessary. The approach is therefore to integrate system solutions into functional clothes with integrated textile sensors. The combination of functional clothes and integrated electronics and on-body processing, is defined as e-textile and gives rise to intelligent biomedical clothes. Systems, designed to be minimally invasive, are based on smart textile technologies, where conductive and piezoresistive materials in the form of fiber and yarn are used to realize clothes, in which knitted fabric sensors and electrodes are distributed and connected to an electronic portable unit. These systems are able to detect, acquire and transmit physiological signals. They are conformable to the human body, and move towards improving the patient's quality of life and their autonomy. These systems are also cost-effective in providing around-the-clock assistance, in helping physicians to monitor for example cardiac patients during periods of rehabilitation, and in addition result in decreased hospitalization time. Finally, by providing direct feedback to the users, they improve their awareness and potentially allow better control of their own condition, while the simultaneous recording of vital signs permits parameter extrapolation and inter-signal elaboration that contributes to produce alert messages and personalized synoptic tables of the patient's health.

Keywords: Wearable, e-textile, healthcare, fabric sensors.

Introduction

A new generation of health care monitoring systems, founded on the exploitation of multidisciplinary research results is emerging. These systems combine the advances of telecommunication, microelectronics and material science to guarantee a continuous remote monitoring of multiple physiological functions, as well as comfort and wearability [1]. Citizens are becoming more and more used in telecommunicating and in managing information, and the idea of a surrounding virtual world is no more an alien concept.

New monitoring systems need to be based on flexible and smart technologies conformable to the human body, to guarantee user's autonomy and higher quality of life and in addition to enhance their motivation and consciousness. One of the stimulating challenges of this approach is the aspiration to acquire the most realistic health status in a "natural" environment and specifically to minimize the interaction between the sensing system and the user activity. For this reason the use of sensing textile materials is gaining more and more attention.

Sensing clothes based on conductive and piezoresistive materials in the form of fibre and yarn, are the common platforms for innovative solutions, where the fabric itself is acting as a sensor and electrode. Textile sensing patterns are distributed and connected to an electronic portable unit. The physiological signals can then be acquired, stored or continuously transmitted to a remote monitoring system. Breathing pattern, electrocardiogram (ECG), electromiogram, activity pattern, temperature, all can be listed as physiological variables that are monitored through such e-textile systems. A Monitoring System for data representation and alert functions, for professional or consumer, needs to be able to create a "friendly environment" by delivering, processing and storing the appropriate information, without interfering with the user's normal daily activity. An example is the WEALTHY system [2], that is targeting patients suffering from heart diseases during and after their rehabilitation and professional workers engaged in extreme environmental conditions.

Textile sensing platforms have also been developed in the frame of the MYHEART project, where different textile sensing models have been designed and realized to fulfill requirements based on 16 different applications, addressing cardiovascular diseases from prevention to chronic phases.

1. E-Textile System Functions

An e-textile system is based on the integration of several functional modules. The main functions of the wearable modules are namely: sensing, conditioning, pre-processing and data transmission.

The sensing textile interface is connected with a portable device where the local processing as well as the communication with the network is performed.

Examples are shown in Figure 1, where one of the latest versions of the WEALTHY prototypes can be seen and in

Figure 2, where an overview of textile sensing prototypes realized in the frame of the MYHEART project is shown.

The WEALTHY prototype is realized with flat-knitting technology, specific yarns are confined in a predefined insulated region by means of intarsia technique. The elasticity is increased by coupling an elastomer to the other yarns during the working process, high elasticity allows freedom of movement and comfort as well as preventing the formation of pleats and crumples. Two types of soft sensors are interfaced [3]: conductive fabric areas used as ECG electrodes as well as respiration sensors (based on skin impedance change) and piezo-resistive fabric used to monitor movements of the articulations of the arms. In the final version of the garment the thorax functional part contains 9 electrodes, all connected with textile insulated tracks.

The right side of Figure 1 details in particular the electrodes and their related integrated connections. The electrode is conductive only on the back side where the fabric is in contact with the body while for the connections, the conductive path is sandwiched between two insulated fabric layers.

Four of the 9 electrodes are used for respiration as depicted in the right of Figure 1; the other 3 electrodes are also visible, namely Einthoven right arm on the left of the figure, Einthoven left arm on the right, V_5 lead, while V_2 lead electrode is used for ECG as well as for the detection of potential for respiration signal measurement. The electrodes used to inject the current IR and IL are the external left and right circled regions. The other two electrodes that are not visible in the window are the right leg on the left of Figure 1 and the reference on the right of the same figure.

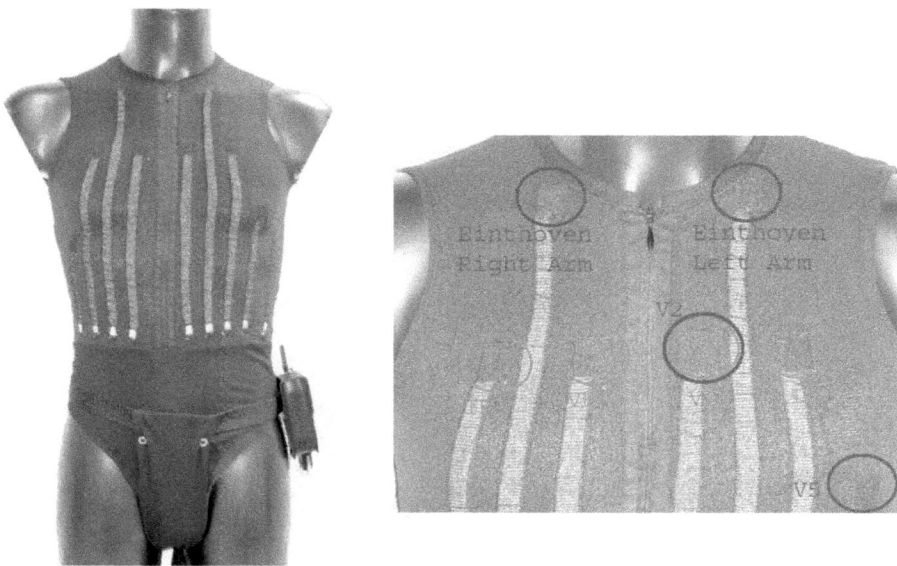

Figure 1. Textile prototypes capable of measuring respiration impedance (I for current injection, V for Voltage measurement) and eletrocardiograms (left and right arms for Einthoven, V2 and V5); one electrode (VL-V2) is used for both respiration and ECG.

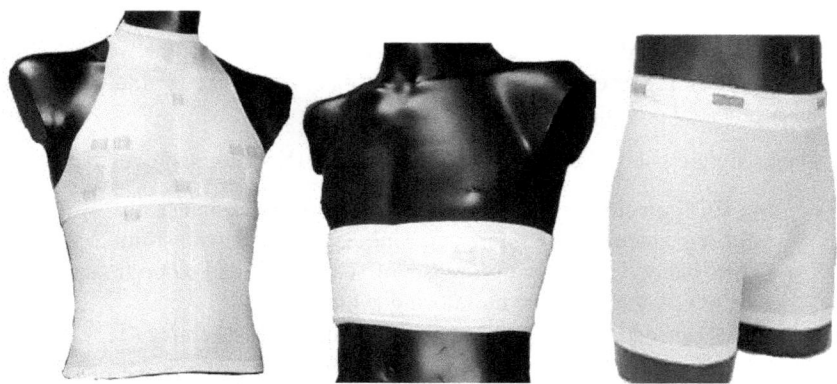

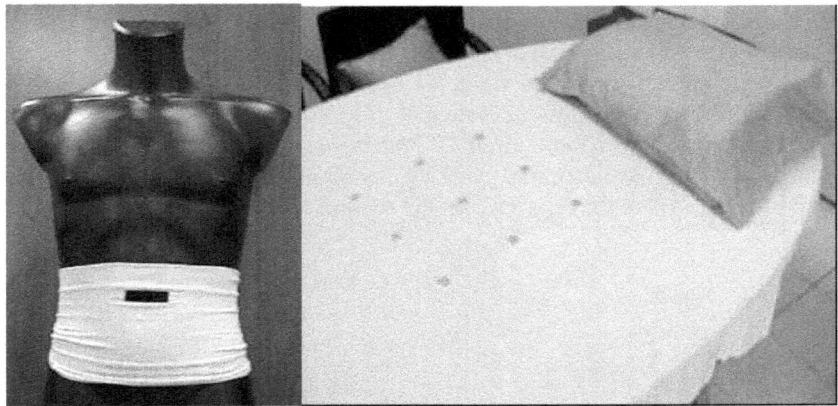

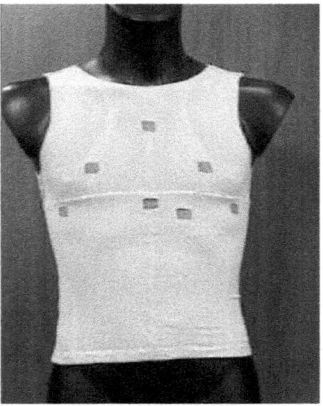

Figure 2. Overview of MYHEART prototypes.

The garment interface is connected with the portable electronic device where the local processing as well as the communication with the network is performed. Most signals are transmitted unprocessed to the Monitoring System where they can be analyzed offline. In order to reduce the required data capacity of the wireless link to the Central Monitoring System, some signals are processed by the portable electronic unit to extract essential parameters.

The complete list of the sensors of the WEALTHY system is given below:

- Six ECG electrodes; lead I, II and III and Precordial leads V_2 and V_5, with right leg electrode as reference. Only one lead is transmitted at a time (for GPRS bandwidth limitation reasons). The ECG lead to be transmitted can be selected remotely by the monitoring center.
- Four electrodes for respiration by impedance measurement.
- Up to four skin temperature sensors (monolithic circuits with an I^2C^{TM} Serial Bus interface).
- One 3D accelerometer (monolithic circuit, integrated in the unit).
- Four piezo-resistive movement sensors.

- SpO_2 (oximetry) from a commercial device (NONIN) (serial interface and power supply provided).

ECG signals are processed on the body, in order to extract parameters at a sampling rate of 250 Hz, while the signal is transmitted at a sampling rate of 125 Hz. Local pre-processing of ECG signals extracts heart rate value and QRS duration. All the other signals are transmitted without local processing.

Off-line processing of parameters, depending on the application, is conducted at the monitoring center, according to the following list:

- Heart rate variability (HRV) [4]
- ST deviation
- T wave area

The final action is to classify recorded parameters to detect an event. Several statistical tools based on a multifunctional analysis, such as PCA or ICA [5], may be used for this purpose.

In order to offer full mobility to the patient or the user, acquired signals are wirelessly transmitted from the portable electronic unit to the remote Monitoring System. The communication is based on TCP/IP (the standard protocol for GPRS communication). All signals are sent in quasi real-time to the remote Monitoring Centre.

The Central Monitoring System comprises the following modules:
- Web Server
- Database Server
- Client Application module
    o Central Control module
    o Doctor's Desktop/Laptop module
    o Doctor's PDA module

All the above modules are able to run on a single computer without the need of dedicated high-end servers.

E-textile platforms give the possibility to monitor and assist patients through a remote medical advice service as well as to give feedback to users. The use of intelligent systems provide physicians with data to detect and manage health risks in a timely fashion, to provide early illness diagnosis, to recommend treatments and prevent further deterioration and, finally, to make confident professional decisions based on objective information all in a reasonably short time.

2. Results

The WEALTHY system is an innovative device able to provide improved health care to users. The integration of multiple parameters and their continuous transmission to a monitoring clinical center makes the system quite unique and different from currently used medical devices.

In Figure 3 an example of simultaneous acquisition of ECG signals obtained from the WEALTHY garment: Einthoven leads D1, D2 and D3 and the precordial leads V_2 and V_5 are visualized. The quality of such signals allows an accurate analysis of possible cardiovascular diseases.

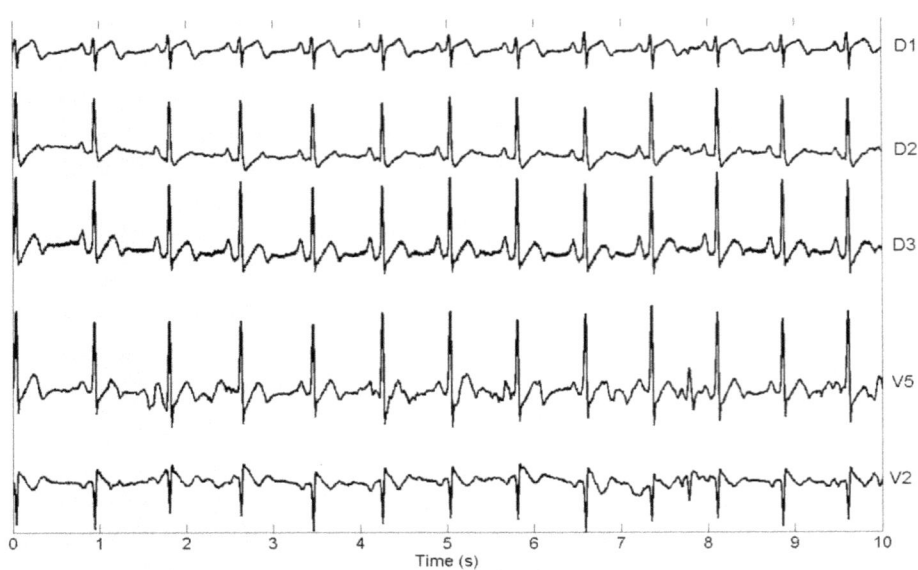

Figure 3. Simultaneous acquisition of ECG leads from the WEALTHY system.

Impedance pneumography technique realised through four electrodes placed in the thorax position allows the extrapolation of several pulmonary parameters, such as respiratory rate and tidal volume.

In Figure 4 an example of a signal obtained by impedance pneumography is shown. It is possible to notice the variation of peak to peak amplitude due to deeper breaths (between 17 to 30 seconds).

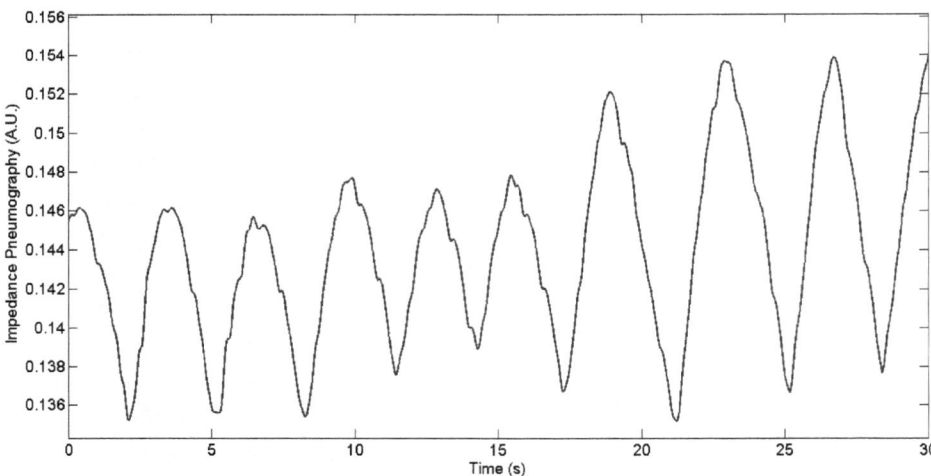

Figure 4. Respiratory activity acquired by impedance pneumography.

3. Discussion

The innovative feature of these systems is the use of conducting and piezoresistive materials in the form of fiber and yarn integrated in a knitted comfortable garment in order to realize sensors, electrodes and tracks.

These elements achieved performance comparable to gold standards [6]. The fabric layout permits the design of an interactive platform that is manufactured in an unconventional way. Nevertheless, a material to be processed with textile machineries must satisfy very strict requirements in terms of mechanical and chemical properties, and for our purposes also in terms of electrical properties.

The potential of using textile facilities is linked to the realization of fibers and yarns suitable to be used in the most sophisticated knitting machines; the fineness, the composition, the mechano-elastic properties of yarns play key roles in this process. The final characteristics of the integrated textile structure are modulated by a series of factors, starting from the material, the combination of yarns, the textile processes, up to the final finishing step. An efficient, wearable and comfortable sensing system is the result of a balance among performance, number and position of the active elements, lightness, comfort and conformability of the final cloth.

The ease of use of such devices provides the possibility of recording physiological variables in a more "natural" environment [7]. This condition may help to identify the influence of the psycho-emotional state of the subject in the performance of a physical activity that is not easily detectable when recording is performed within a protected (medical) environment.

The possibility of simultaneously recording different cardiopulmonary signals provides an integrated view of normal and abnormal patterns of activity and respiratory parameters which could be otherwise impossible to be detected by recording each signal at different times. In addition, the same set of sensors will yield a wide series of respiratory indexes useful for diagnosing several clinical conditions affecting respiratory dynamics.

These new integrated knitted systems enable applications extending even beyond the clinical area and open new possible applications in sport, ergonomics and monitoring operators exposed to harsh or risky conditions (firemen, soldiers etc.).

4. Conclusions

The innovative approach of this work is based on the use of standard textile industrial processes to realize the sensing elements. Transduction functions are implemented in the same knitted system, where movements and vital signs are converted into readable signals, which can be acquired and transmitted.

In these systems, electrodes and bus structures are integrated in textile material, making it possible to perform normal daily activities while the user's clinical status is monitored by a specialist, without any discomfort.

Acknowledgment

The authors would like to thank the European Commission and all partners involved in both projects: WEALTHY IST2001-37778 and MYHEART IST 2002-507816, in particular CSEM responsible for the portable electronic units.

References

[1] S. Park, and S. Jayaraman, "Enhancing the quality of life through wearable technology," *IEEE Engineering in Medicine and Biology Magazine,* vol.22, No.3, pp.41-48, May-June 2003.

[2] R. Paradiso, G. Loriga and N. Taccini, "A Wearable Health Care System Based on Knitted Integrated Sensors", IEEE TITB, to be published.

[3] R. Paradiso, "Tessuto in maglia per il monitoraggio di segnali vitali", Italian Patent N. FI2003A000308, December 3, 2003..

[4] Task Force of the European Society of Cardiology and the North America Society of Pacing and Electrophysiology, "Heart rate variability standards of measurement, physiological interpretation and clinical use" *Circulation* 93(5): pp.1043-65, 1996

[5] A. Hyvarinen, J. Karhunen and E. Oja, 'Independent Component Analysis', J. Wiley &Sons, New York, 2001

[6] E. P. Scilingo, A. Gemignani, R. Paradiso, N. Taccini, B. Ghelarducci, and D. De Rossi, (2004) "Sensing Fabrics for Monitoring Physiological and Biomechanical Variables," IEEE TITB, to be published.

[7] D. Franchi, A. Belardinelli, G. Palagi, A. Ripoli, and R. Bedini, "New telemedicine approach to the dynamic ECG and other biological signals ambulatory monitoring" *Computers in Cardiology,*vol.25, pp.213-216. 1998.

Personalised Health Management Systems
C.D. Nugent et al. (Eds.)
IOS Press, 2005

Electroactive Fabrics for Distributed, Comfortable and Interactive Systems

Federico Lorussi[1,2], Alessandro Tognetti[1], Mario Tesconi[1], Giuseppe Zupone[1],
Raphael Bartalesi[1] and Danilo De Rossi[1,2]

[1]*Interdepartemental Research Centre "E.Piaggio", University of Pisa, Via Diotisalvi 2,
Pisa, Italy*
[2]*Information Engineering Department, University of Pisa, Via Caruso 2, Pisa, Italy*

Abstract. Monitoring body kinematics has fundamental relevance in several biological and technical disciplines. In particular the possibility to know the posture exactly may furnish a main aid in rehabilitation topics. In the present work a collection of innovative and unobtrusive garments able to detect the posture and the movement of the human body are introduced. This paper deals with the design, the development and the realization of sensing garments, from the characterization of innovative comfortable and spreadable sensors to the methodologies employed to gather information on the posture and movement. Several new algorithms devoted to the device operation are presented and tested. Data derived from the sensing garment are analyzed and compared with the data derived from a traditional movement tracking system.

Keywords. Body kinematics, Sensorised garments, Rehabilitation.

Introduction

This work deals with the development of innovative measuring systems devoted to the human movement analysis. Our main aim is to provide a valid, alternative and comfortable system useful in several fields; rehabilitation areas, sport disciplines and multimedia applications.

The analysis of human movement is generally performed by measuring kinematic variables of anatomic segments by employing accelerometers, electrogoniometers, electromagnetic sensors or cameras integrated in finer equipment such as stereophotogrammetric systems. Several disadvantages in remote rehabilitation tasks derive from the use of these technologies which are mainly applied in the realization of robotics or mechatronics machines (such as MIME or MIT-MANUS [1]). They often result in invasive and complex solutions which are unable to satisfy safety requirements for the presence of mechanical parts while they move. In the literature, several studies are devoted to realize electric devices with properties of high wearability [2, 3]. The main drawbacks of wearable sensing systems available on the market are their weight, the rigidity of the fabric which they are made of, the dimension of the sensors used, and all the other properties which make them obtrusive. In particular, conventional sensors often require the application of complex and uncomfortable mechanical plugs in order to position the sensors on garments.

In the present paper, we focused our efforts on the realization of new systems for the measurement of the human body kinematic variables by means of sensorized garments such as an Upper Limb Kinesthetic Garment (ULKG), a Sensing glove, a Sensorized Knee Band and a Catsuit, as shown in Figure 1.

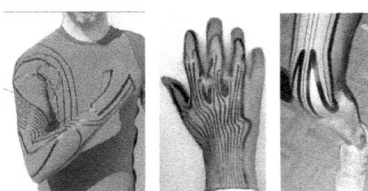

Figure 1. The sensing garments.

Lightness, adherence and elasticity have been privileged in the system realization as fundamental requirements for their unobtrusivity. These guidelines have led us to choose an elastic fabric (Lycra) to manufacture them as sensorized garments. In order to equip the lycra garments with a sensing apparatus, sensors have been spread on the fabric by employing an electrically conductive elastomer (CE). CE deposition does not change the mechanical characteristics of the fabric. It preserves the wearability of the garments and it confers to the fabric piezoresistive properties related to mechanical solicitations. Furthermore, by using this technology, both sensors and interconnection wires can be smeared by using the same material in a single printing and manufacturing process. This is a real improvement in terms of comfort performed by the device because no metallic wires are necessary to interconnect sensors or to connect them to the electronic acquisition and processing unit. In this way no rigid constraints are present and movements are unbounded.

1. Wearable Sensors

CE composites show piezoresistive properties when a deformation is applied and can be integrated into fabric or other flexible substrate to be employed as strain sensors. Integrated CE sensors obtained in this way may be used in posture and movement analysis by realizing wearable kinesthetic interfaces [4]. The CE we used is a commercial product by WACKER Ltd (Elastosil LR 3162 A/B) [5] and it consists of a mixture containing graphite and silicon rubber. WACKER Ltd guarantees the nontoxicity of the product that, after the vulcanization, can be employed in medical and pharmaceutical applications.

In the realization of the sensorised garment, a solution of Elastosil and trichloroethylene is smeared on a lycra substrate previously covered by an adhesive mask. The mask has been designed according to the desired topology of the sensor network and cut by a laser milling machine. After the CE deposition, the mask is removed and the treated fabric is placed in an oven at a temperature of $130°C$ to speed up the cross-linking process of the mixture.

An analysis of the electrical, mechanical and thermal transduction properties and aging of the fabric has been executed [3]. In terms of quasi-static characterization, a sample of 5mm in width shows an unstretched electrical resistance of about 1k per cm, and its gauge factor (GF) is about 2.8. GF can be expressed as in equation 1;

$$GF = \frac{l(R - R_0)}{R(l - l_0)} \qquad (1)$$

where R is the electrical resistance, l is the actual length, R_0 is the electrical resistance corresponding to l_0 which represents the rest length of the specimen. The temperature coefficient ratio is $0.08K^{-1}$. Capacity effects exhibited by the sample are negligible up to 100MHz. A wide and exhaustive characterization of the physical and piezoresistive dynamical properties of CE sensors, can be found in [6] where all these issues have been completely addressed.

2. Garment Electrical Model and Electronic Acquisition Techniques

An example of a sensorized prototype, realized by using an mask, is shown in Figure 2. The bold black track represents the set of sensors connected in series (S_i), and covers the main joints of the upper limb (shoulder, elbow and wrist). The thin tracks (R_i) represent the connection between the sensor set and the electronic acquisition system.

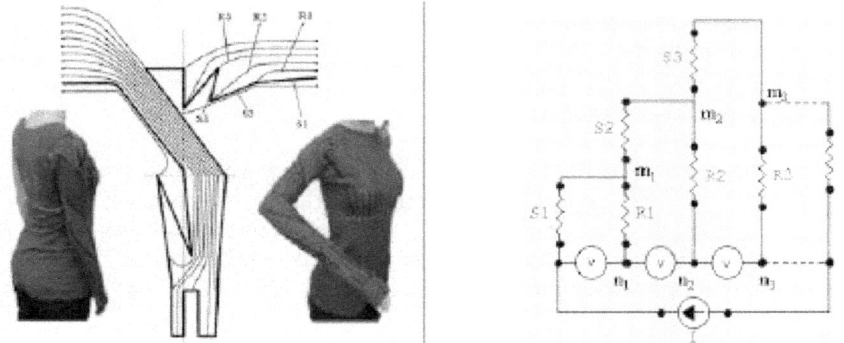

Figure 2. Mask for the realization of the ULKG prototype and electronic reading scheme.

Since the thin tracks are made of the same piezoresitive CE mixture, they undergo a non-negligible (and unknown) change in their resistance when the upper limb moves. Therefore the analog front-end of the electronic unit is designed to compensate this resistance variation. In Figure 2 the electric schematic is also reported. While a generator supplies the series of sensors S_i with a constant current I, the acquisition system has been provided by a high input impedance stage realized by instrumentation amplifiers and represented in Figure 2 by the set of voltmeters. Thanks to this configuration, only a small amount of current flows through the connecting wires, which have resistance values R_i, and so the voltages which fall on R_i are negligible if the current I is big enough. In conclusion, the voltages measured by the instrumentation amplifiers are equal to the voltages which fall on the S_i that is related to the resistances of the sensors. In this way, the thin galley proofs perfectly substitute the traditional metallic wires and a sensor, consisting in a segment of the bold track between two thin tracks, can be smeared in any position to detect the movements of a certain joint.

3. The Wearable Sensing Garment

3.1. The Upper Limb Sensing Garment (ULKG)

The ULKG is a new system for the measurement of the human upper limb kinematic variables. ULKG is under testing in post-stroke patients' rehabilitation. The main institution involved in the testing of the system to helpfully employ it in a medical context is the S.Maugeri Foundation, in Pavia, Italy. This unit is responsible for the drawing up of a post-stroke rehabilitation protocol for hemiplegic patients according to the guideline contained in [7].

Using the ULKG, it is possible to detect if two postures are the same or not with a certain tolerance, and it is possible to record a certain set of postures coded by the status of the sensors. Moreover, movements can be recorded as the transition from one posture to another, and they are coded by the evolution of the sensor values. In particular, we have tested this capability on a set of functional relevant postures which have been related to the corresponding configurations in the model represented by the avatar. After having stored all the data concerning fifty different postures in the upper limb workspace, the same postures recorded again. An ad-hoc software system devoted to recognize recorded postures has been developed. The software is able to:

i)   record a set of defined postures of the upper limb in a calibration phase,
ii) recognize the recorded postures during the user's movements and
iii) represent the movement by using a graphical representation given by the avatar as shown in Figure 3. The system recognized 100% of the postures recorded, and no further re-calibration has been necessary even if the ULKG has been removed and re-worn.

3.2. Glove for Gesture Recognition

We have realized a second sensing garment in a glove made of Lycra which satisfies the requirements of lightness, elasticity and adherence.

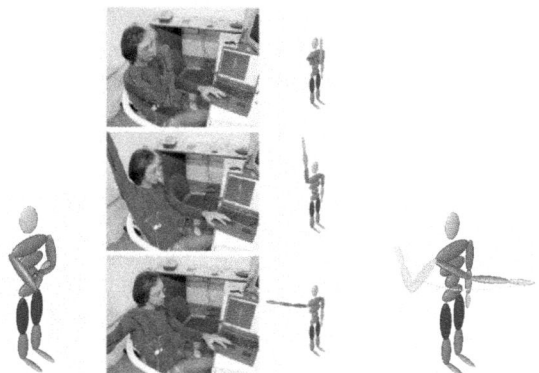

Figure 3. Avatar and Posture recognition trials.

We integrated sensors into a glove as shown in Figure 4 which were linked to an electronic unit which treats the pre-filtered obtained data.

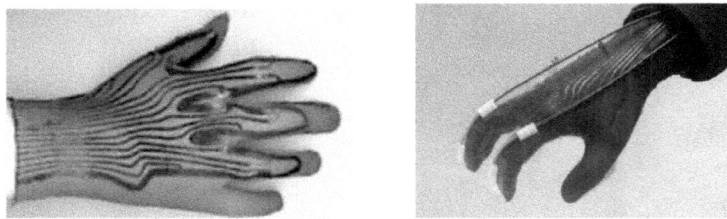

Figure 4. The sensorised glove and its calibration.

The glove has demonstrated good capabilities of repeatability, in detecting postures, even if it is removed from the hand and re-worn (by the same subject). It has been possible to detect if two postures are the same or not, and it has been possible to record a certain set of postures coded by the status of the sensors. As for the ULKG, movements have been recorded as transitions from one posture to another. In particular, we have tested this capability on a set of functionally relevant postures, the basic hand grip. An ad-hoc software system devoted to recognize the recorded hand posture has been developed. Although this working mode for the glove is quite simple, it seems to be very promising for several applications in rehabilitation therapies and medicine. Some of the basic positions acquired during the posture recorder mode can be used to construct a continuous function which maps position into sensor values. This map, obtained as an interpolation of the discrete function which recognizes recorded posture, can be used to detect any position of the hand, even if it has never been told. In fact, the identification algorithm is able to construct a model of the hand expressed in terms of sensor values. If the basic position recorded is associated to a set of angle deviations for the joints of the hand, for example by using in a calibration phase a set of electrogoniometers (Figure 4), the inversion algorithm reconstructs the position (in terms of angles) which have never been assumed by the subject.

The glove, used as a posture recorder, is required to verify only the hypothesis of repeatability. In the test we have performed (on a set of 32 different postures, the basic grip and the sign of the American sign language), the glove has recognized 100% of the postures previously recorded if it was not removed from the hand, and 98% when it has been re-worn. The percentage increases to 100% if the system is re-adjusted when the first error occurs. The Sensing Glove has also been used as a PC mouse and it has been possible to control a 2D PC pointer. Flexion-extension of forefinger or of the thumb codify vertical movements while abduction-adduction-codify horizontal movements of the pointer in a PC screen. The glove when used as a mouse pointer can be directly connected to a joystick plug, so it is compatible with most PCs without the need of any other electronic acquisition device. This device can be utilized in working environments for subjects with pathologies which bound upper limb mobility.

3.3. The Sensing Knee Sleeve

The knee-sleeve has been designed and realized in order to investigate the knee joint in sport applications. The knee is a very stressed joint and it is subjected to continuous efforts in all sporting disciplines. The knee-sleeve has been realized following an anatomical and bio-mechanical study of the knee in order to externally reproduce the position of its 4 mean ligaments. Figure 5 shows the knee-band and the relative mask.

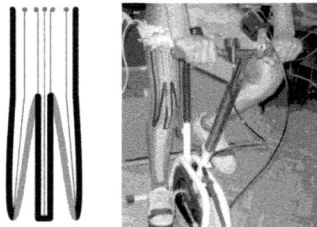

Figure 5. Knee-band and the relative mask.

The reliability of the system has been verified using Biometrics electrogoniometers, that have an accuracy of +/- 2°. The results obtained following the analysis of the flex-extension movement have been satisfactory and are shown in Figure 6, where the violet and the blue lines point out the angles relieved by the knee-band and the ones read by the electrogoniometers respectively. A wireless acquisition device has been realized in order to monitor the gesture of a subject and preserve their freedom of movement. This allows an athlete to use it in many sport disciplines that often require a large space for the execution of the characteristic movements. This device can be used for knee stability tests (ligaments status evaluation) and for injury prevention and rehabilitation in soccer, providing an instrument for the analysis of the technical gesture. A similar device has been developed by CSIRO, Au [8].

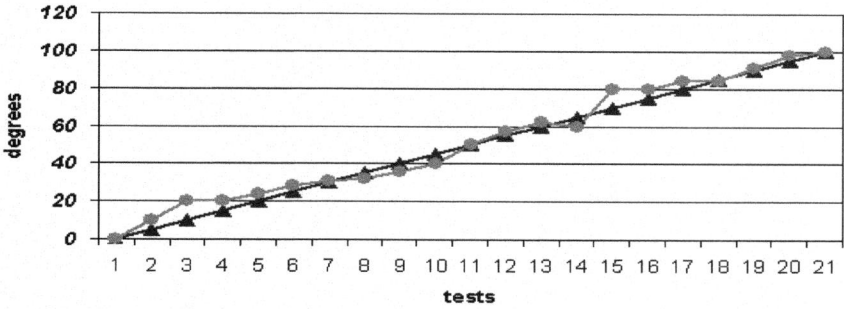

Figure 6. Graph tests vs degrees.

3.4. The Catsuit

The Catsuit is an interactive and personalized system for the management of the training of sporting techniques from a technical and tactical point of view. It has been studied for the monitoring of the golf swing, but it is applicable to many other disciplines. The system consists of a wearable sensorised catsuit controlled by a portable control system able to evaluate and improve the athlete and neophyte performances. The system can be used in any common fitness activity, and can be employed as a useful tool in teaching the basic technical gestures in various disciplines. It is able to relieve the posture and the incorrect gesture during particular movements. This information can be used to evaluate and correct the necessary motor scheme for a particular action. In addition it can be used either to improve and refine the athletic gesture or to plan a specific course of training in order to solve any technical and physical problems during high levels of activities. In the Figure 7 the positioning of the sensors and the relative mask for the sensorised catsuit are presented.

4. Conclusions

In this work a collection of sensorised garments for the human body gesture, posture and movement evaluation has been presented. The main advantage offered by these prototypes is the possibility of wearing them for long periods and being monitored without discomfort. Several issues, deriving from the employment of the new technology which has consented the realization of these unobtrusive devices have been addressed. Moreover, it has been pointed out that the use of these sensorised garments as valid alternative and comfortable instrumentation are applicable in several rehabilitation areas, in sport disciplines and in multimedia applications.

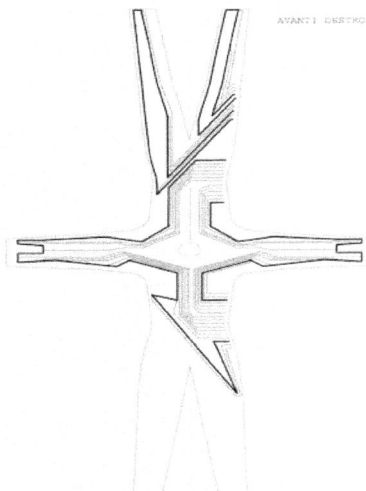

Figure 7. Positioning of the sensors and the relative mask for the sensorised catsuit.

Acknowledgements

This research has been funded by the European Commission through MyHeart project - IST 507816, DARPA and ONR-IFO through NICOP grant N00014-01-1-0280, Pr N 01PR04487-00.

References

[1]   Krebs HI, Ferraro M, Buerger SP, Newbery MJ, Makiyama A, Sandmann M, Lynch D, Volpe BT, Hogan N: Rehabilitation robotics: pilot trial of a spatial extension for MIT-Manus. *Journal of NeuroEngineering and Rehabilitation* 2004, **1**(5).
[2]   Post ER, Orth M, Russo PR, Gershenfeld N: Design and fabrication of textile-based computing. IBM System Journal 2000, 39(34).
[3]   Scilingo EP, Lorussi F, Mazzoldi A, De Rossi D: Sensing Fabrics forWearable Kinaesthetic-Like Systems. IEEE Sensors Journal 2003, 3(4):460–467.
[4]   Lorussi F, RocchiaW, Scilingo EP, Tognetti A, De Rossi D:Wearable Redundant Fabric-Based Sensors Arrays for Reconstruction of Body Segment Posture. IEEE Sensors Journal 2004, 4(6):807–818.
[5]   Elastosil LR3162[http://www.wacker.com].
[6]   A.Tognetti, F.Lorussi, M.Tesconi, D. De Rossi, "Strain sensing fabric characterization", Third IEEE International Conference on Sensors, Vienna, Austria, October 24-27, 2004.
[7]   The Stroke Prevention and Educational Awareness Diffusion (SPREAD) Collaboration.
[8]   http://www.csiro.au/index.asp?type=mediaRelease&id=prkneesleeve&stylesheet=mediaRelease

Personalised Health Management Systems
C.D. Nugent et al. (Eds.)
IOS Press, 2005

Point of Care Biomedical Sensors

J.A.D McLAUGHLIN
NIBEC and NRI
University of Ulster, Newtownabbey, Co. Antrim, Northern Ireland, BT37 OQB

Abstract. With the development of critical areas of interdisciplinary research, scientists will lead to an enhanced understanding and control of the key processing stages involved in the design and manufacture of sensor-and electrode-based micro-devices such as micro total analysis systems (µTAS), bio-chips, bio-arrays and DNA sensors. It is anticipated that this fundamental work will lead to tangible technology transfer in the areas of blood analysis, cardiac enzyme detectors, liver and renal function, infectious diseases, gene disorders, etc. These will obviously have major benefits to healthcare delivery. The development of miniaturised, integrated sensor/electrode-based devices are revolutionising both the delivery of health care. In this paper, some of the most exciting research themes in these areas are identified, as well as novel underpinning fabrication technologies and transduction principles, which should make future advances possible.

Keywords: Biomedical Sensor, Device Fabrication, Point of Care.

Introduction

Present trends in Biomedicine include exciting developments in what have come to be known as *'Point-of-Care Medicine'*. Historically, most laboratory testing has been carried out in a remote, centralised laboratory and hence involves considerable time, manpower and expense. Recently, there has been a rapid shift towards near-patient or 'point-of-care' testing of key analytes where a rapid 'turn-around' time is essential in the successful management of critically ill patients, especially during open-heart surgery [1]. Many advantages in this approach have been reported as it is progressively being introduced into a wide range of 'non-life-threatening', patient monitoring applications. Sample volumes are generally very small and test results may be acted upon immediately, thus facilitating on-going management of a chronic disease. As there is no need to transport the specimen for remote testing, there is a reduced biohazard and practically no possibility of mix-ups between patients' results [2]. Devices successfully introduced to the market include those of I-STAT and SenDx (recently bought over by Radiometer). These miniaturised laboratory systems are based on thickfilm sensor technology, as shown in Figure 1 [3].

These thick film-based sensor systems incorporate an array of individually designed sensors capable of detecting specific anayltes such as pH, pCO2, pO2, Na+, K+, iCa++ and haematocrit from whole blood. The individual sensors are generally amperometric potentiometric or conductometric based with ion-selective membranes.

The mini array is equipped with pre-packaged calibrating reagent solutions, integral heating element and temperature sensor. A small sample of blood, for example, flows past the sensors and all the parameters are measured in less than 60 seconds.

Thick film technology has proved very successful [4], however, for its advantages to be fully exploited, there is a need to integrate treatment delivery with analyte detection [5, 6].

The I-STAT(TM) analyser is a miniaturised, portable, hand-held chemistry analyser which integrates semiconductor manufacturing process technology with well defined electrochemical principles, thus resulting in the production of micro-miniaturised sensors with highly reproducible characteristics. Silicon-type microfabrication utilising high quality materials that exhibit exceptional stability allows consistent reproducibility in a high-volume manufacturing environment. Once testing is complete, the patient data is stored automatically and can be recalled later, printed and/or transferred electronically to the hospital's information systems using infrared.

The University of Ulster have pioneered the development of portable vital signs monitoring systems which have been successfully commercialised by Shahal Medical services and Phillips Medical. The patient subscriber is provided with a CardioBeeper® trans-telephonic ECG transmitter and the LidoPen® lidocaine auto-injector. 24 hours a day, subscribers can call the monitoring centre and using any telephone or cellular phone, they can transmit a full 12 lead ECG to the dedicated monitoring centre, staffed by nurses under physician supervision, for the purpose of remote real time diagnosis of arrhythmia, ischaemia, and myocardial infacrtion.

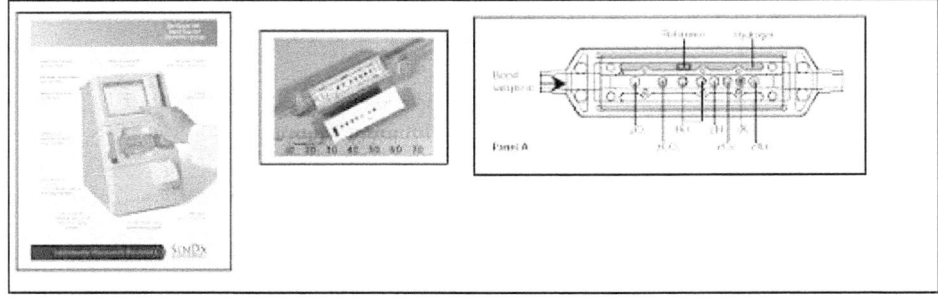

Figure 1. Sen Dx Blood Gas and Electrolyte Sensing System.

Several groups are presently developing the concept of intelligent wearable monitoring sensor systems. This approach has the potential to substantially change the provision of health and health care services for large population groups, e.g. those suffering from chronic diseases (such as cardiovascular, diabetes, respiratory and neurological disorders), the elderly with specific needs, fire fighters, emergency workers and the military. At present, these wearable systems exist in pre-commercial states or are just entering commercial stage. Examples of such systems are Mamagoose-Pyjama for the detection of Sudden Infant Death Syndrome (Verhaert, Belgium), and LifeShirt-Continuous Ambulatory Monitoring (VivoMetrics, USA). Other research and development activities in real time personal care wearable systems are ongoing in Europe and world-wide, e.g. AMON (Wrist Telemedical Monitor) and Lifebelt (wearable device for health monitoring during pregnancy) currently funded by the IST (Information Society Technologies) programme of the EC.

In certain instances, it may be desirable to further extend the 'point-of-care' monitoring concept and implant the sensor in the patient, temporarily at present and permanently in the future. NIBEC at the University of Ulster have been involved in several European research programs developing sensor arrays for temporary implanting into the heart during open heart surgery or during organ transport and transplant (Figure 2). The MICROCARD device consists of a thin multisensor silicon needle for simultaneous measurement of transmural changes in the myocardial tissue impedance, extracellular K+ concentration and pH induced by acute myocardial ischaemia. The device is to be used in the early detection of myocardial ischaemia during cardiac surgery. In MICROTRANS a multifunctional silicon microprobe with integrated microsensors is implanted in the organ during transportation and key parameters (pH, [K+], temperature and impedance) are monitored continuously to ensure organ viability.

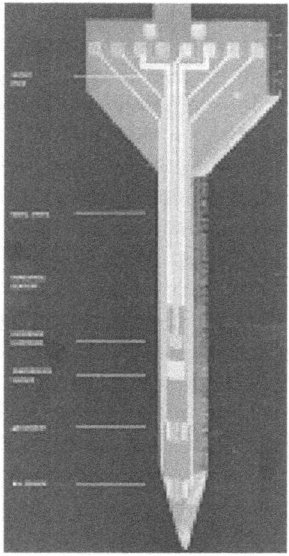

Figure 2. UU Micromachined Electrode needle.

1. The DNA chip , Lab-On Chip and Protein Chip

The current market for the DNA chip [7], Lab-on chip and protein Chip [8] is approximately $300M with the platform technology playing a major role in other markets. Analysts expect it to grow by approximately 50% a year through to 2005 [11]. Not only can Micro-technologies fuel biomedical product innovations (thus improving existing products through 'added-value') but, most exciting of all, can lead to totally new concepts, solutions and hence novel device types [9, 10].

There has been a shift in emphasis from an early preoccupation with bioreagent immobilisation and chemistry to an effort towards integration of micro 'total analysis systems' (µTAS). Presently, there is much interest in enhanced performance antibody-and DNA-based sensors although improvements may also be achieved with engineered enzyme-based devices. Such devices offer considerable promise for obtaining the sequence-specific information in a faster, simpler and cheaper manner compared to traditional hybridisation assays. The rapid advances in DNA microarray and biosensor technologies have enabled applications ranging from genetic testing to gene expression and drug discovery. Further miniaturisation, particularly of the support instrumentation, should lead to hand-held DNA analysers, for example [9]. The coupling of fundamental biological and chemical sciences with technological advances in the fields of micromachining and microfabrication should lead to even more powerful devices that will accelerate the realisation of large-scale genetic testing. A wide range of new gene chips and DNA biosensors are thus expected to reach the market over the coming years. With the completion of the human genome project, we are at the beginning of a revolution in genetic analysis, leading to the development of vital tests and the critical assessment of medical treatments.

The long term move away move from bioaffinity and biocatalytic biosensors to nucleic acid based DNA sensors, where recognition layers can be readily synthesised and regenerated for multiple use, is witnessing huge interest. Hybridisation biosensors rely on the immobilisation of a single–stranded DNA probe onto a transducer surface. The duplex formation can be detected following the association of an appropriate hybridisation indicator or through other changes accrued from the binding event. Important aspects of developing these sensor types include surface chemistry, biochemistry, transducer technology (i.e. optical, electrical or mass sensitive), etc.

DNA microarrays/biochips/gene chips offer great potential for highly accurate, miniaturised and rapid multiplex analysis of nucleic acid samples, leading to diagnosis of diseases, infectious agents, drug screening and measurement of gene expression. Full sample processing at point-of-care will be the ultimate goal. It is envisaged that this will involve 'credit card' size integration of sample preparation, DNA extraction, amplification, hybridisation, microfluidics and DNA array detection - known as 'Lab on chip'. New evolving fabrication techniques being studied for this purpose include micro-sized pumps, heaters, valves, channels, electrodes etc. Lawrence Livermore National Laboratories and Hewlett Packard have already developed PCR chips. Nanogen have successfully demonstrated several of the steps involved in the fabrication of a complete Lab on Chip module.

2. Transduction Techniques

An increasing number of transduction techniques are available to potentially suit the scale, cost and accuracy requirements of the sensing system. Surface plasmon resonance (SPR), Impedimetry, Fluorescence based Biochemistry, Colourimetry, SAW, Micro-balance etc., are all examples of technologies that have been demonstrated, to some extent at least, to work at device level although in some cases further planarisation and integration with electronics and sample handling are needed to allow new sensor markets to develop.

Two particularly promising transduction techniques for biomedical monitoring include Surface Plasmon Resonance and Impedance sensing. The next two sections provide some details on how the miniaturisation of the techniques will lead to new biomedical sensors.

3. Surface Plasmon Resonance

Recent developments in SPR technology have made this transduction technique very desirable for a wide range of biosensing applications, particularly those of affinity determination and real time immunoassays [14, 15, 17]. The technique lends itself to the detection of very small concentrations of analyte and is specific only to reactions occurring at the sensor surface. SPR is a physical process that can occur when plane-polarised light hits a metallic film under total internal reflection (TIR) conditions. A prism is typically coated with a thin gold film on the reflection site. When the energy of the photon electrical field is just right it can interact with the free electron constellations in the gold surface. The incident light photons are absorbed and converted into surface plasmons. Resonance occurs when the momentum of incoming light is equal to the momentum of the plasmons (momentum resonance). In TIR, the reflected photons create an electric field on the opposite site of the interface. The plasmons create a comparable field that extends into the medium on either side of the film. This field is called the evanescent wave because it decays with distance. The binding of biomolecules results in the change of the refractive index on the film, which is measured as a change in reflected light. The change in refractive index on the surface is linearly related to the amount of molecules bound.

SPR is a powerful technique to measure biomolecular interactions in real-time in a label free environment [16, 19]. While one of the interactants is immobilised to the sensor surface, the other are free in solution and passed over the surface. Association and dissociation is measured and kinetic rate constants can be determined. This technique is not limited to protein-protein interactions but all kind of interactions between molecules can be measured. Examples are DNA-protein, lipid protein and protein - plastic surfaces etc. [20].

The gold sensor chip surface has already proved to be suitable for use as a biosensor surface and covalent bonding of alkanthiol molecules onto the gold surface has been successfully achieved in the form of a self-assembled monolayer. This layer forms an effective insulating substrate for biomolecule attachment and the basic biosensor structure. It has been observed that the self-assembly occurs effectively only on the <111> oriented gold surface using AFM/STM techniques. The effect of deposition processing on crystallographic orientation of the grain structure is therefore of fundamental importance to such a technique and thus, the growth processes and material properties of all the deposited thin film layers which make up the sensor.

In SPR biosensors, transduction is achieved by the modification of the refractive index of the recognition layer [12]. Such physical change correlates directly with the molecular recognition event. In the case of an immunosensing device, the biochemical modification consists on the couplage between an antibody and its target analyte [19, 22]. Thus, the design of the recognition layer implies the immobilisation of antibodies either in a bulk material or in a molecular monolayer. In each case, antibodies must be accessible to their target molecule, thus immobilisation materials should be sufficiently porous. However, due to the small size of antibodies, physical bulk immobilisation is not appropriate. Moreover, the orientation and the specificity of antibodies must be preserved during immobilisation, thus cross-linking via bi-functional agents is inappropriate. The immobilisation techniques mainly used in SPR are physical adsorption (which has the drawback of mechanical instability) and covalent binding. This binding should be processed either in a bulk 3D matrix or in monolayer structures. In any case, this implies a specific derivation of antibodies [21].

Bulk immobilisation and covalent grafting of antibodies at gold surfaces is also key to the sensitivity of a device. Bulk immobilisation is obtained using hydrogel materials adsorbed on hydrophobic gold film modified by alkane thiol self-assembled monolayers. Dextran gels including grafting sites have been used for the antibodies. This technique presents the advantage of simplicity and accessibility of the antibodies in the matrix. Furthermore, gold films could be reusable after a simple dissolution of the gel layer. Another method of interest deals with the functionalisation of electropolymerisable monomers such as pyrrole with an antibody. In this case, the coating process becomes selective (electrochemical formation of a polymer film at an electrode surface) and enables the design of multi-sensor arrays.

Monolayer assemblies are of interest because, contrary to bulk immobilisation, antibodies could be oriented. Thus, antibodies could be directly grafted onto gold surfaces using S-H bounds. Another possibility consists of the "hydrophobisation" of gold surfaces, using alkanethiol monolayers for example, followed by the coating of an amphiphilic antibody monolayer (antibody modified by an hydrophobic alkyl chain).

4. Impedimetric Sensors

Over the past few years there has been a rapid growth in publications on Impedimetric sensors, especial in the areas of microbial monitoring and nano-scaled affinity based biosensors for both DNA- and immuno-sensing applications. Impedance transduction is highly suited to modern planar technologies as it avoids the problem of fabricating the reference electrode required in potentiometric sensing. No internal reference solution is required and the electrodes are relatively simple and low cost to make.

In cellular impedimetric sensing the attachment and spreading behaviour of cells can be an important parameter, easily detected using impedance-based sensors, which has been used to distinguish between cancerous and non-cancerous tissues. Normal cells need to be attached to a surface before they grow whereas cancerous cells usually can grow and produce freely in a medium without being attached to any substrate or surface. Obviously, impedance measurements involving cancerous and non-cancerous cells will differ significantly due to the latter's attachment and spread on the measurement electrode surface. This is a very simple and effective technique with a wide range of uses.

Impedimetric biosensors are being developed to detect affinity binding of target biomolecular structures such as antigens or DNA to a sensor surface as a result of the electric field between the electrodes changing due to the presence of the targeted biomolecule.

As impedimetric sensing avoids the need of labelling the target, it is an attractive direct method of biosensing. Nano-scaled electrodes detect events occurring on or in close proximity to the electrode surfaces. Scaling down the dimensions of electrochemical detectors offers new possibilities in terms of sensitivity and signal to background discrimination.

Electrical impedance is a measure of how electricity travels through a given (bio)material. A current or voltage is applied via electrodes to the material, the resultant voltage or current measured and the impedance calculated over a range of frequencies. Impedance measurements can reveal information on the structure of the sample and/or the processes that occur at the electrode-sample interface or in the bulk of the sample. Various designs and arrangements of electrodes, as well as choice of the applied signal frequency range and experimental protocol can be set so as to selectively highlight interfacial or bulk properties of interest [23].

Over the past few years there has been a rapid growth in publications on Impedimetric sensors, especially in the areas of microbial monitoring and nanoscaled, affinity-based biosensors for both DNA- and immuno-sensing applications [24; 25]. Whilst it is gratifying to note the increased appreciation of the numerous advantages associated with Impedimetric sensing, it is disconcerting to discover widespread lack of understanding of the limitations of the technique, especially when misused or misinterpreted. Errors typically made include the use of inappropriate electrode materials, electrode designs and layout, frequency range of study, experimental protocol and equivalent circuit model [26, 27]. Much of what is published is, at best, less than optimal. Often, what is being reported is largely recording artefact.

Contrary to the apparent widespread assumption, 'there is more to electrodes than making them smaller and conductive'. The associated science has to be developed if meaningful results are to be obtained. More complete investigations are required of the above aspects of electrode/impedance technology to enable the full exploitation of this 'new' transduction principle in the areas of cellular and biomolecular monitoring. One key area of study will be surface topography effects on electrode impedances. As electrode area decreases its impedance increases, making accurate measurements difficult – especially in the case of micro/nano sensors. Increasing surface porosity, for a given area, decreases electrode interface impedance and minimises these problems [28]. Electrode fabrication, surface modification and surface characterisation techniques are therefore of great importance if meaningful results are to be obtained.

In cellular sensing the attachment and spreading behaviour of cells is being used to distinguish between cancerous and non-cancerous tissues [29, 30]. Impedance measurements involving these cells are found to differ significantly due to the latter's attachment and spread on the measurement electrode surface. This very simple technique has been shown to be effective and potentially has a wide range of uses, including studies of cell growth, motility and migration.

Although the technique already exists, it is still in its infancy and development of the sensing technique will greatly enhance the sensor's sensitivity, range of applications, ease of manufacture and integration into miniaturised 'SMART' systems. A more appropriate '3-electrode' technique is being researched at UU along with the use of multifrequency Electrical Impedance Spectroscopy, possibly enabling the 'finger-printing' of the cells involved. Micro/nano sensor fabrication will enable wide spread use of the technique in a range of exciting applications such as the study of cell proliferation (and rate of) on an impedimetric electrode surface.

Another pioneering area for cellular impedimetric sensing is in the use of Electrical Impedance Spectroscopy (EIS) to monitor the changes in cells during Low-Voltage Electroporation (LVEP). LVEP is an exiting new technique that overcomes the major deficiency of existing electroporation techniques, low cell survival, and has successfully transfected plasmids into mammalian cells [31]. EIS will be used to provide a wealth of information on the LVEP processes as well as forming an essential part of the system's feedback and control. The key to success in this area is electrode micro/nano-fabrication, surface science and cellular Impedance characterisation.

Engineers continue to advance the area of Micro/Nano-scale Impedimetric immuno- and geno-sensors as there is an identified need for miniature, sensitive and easy-to-use devices. One area of great interest is the development of novel nanoscaled impedimetric affinity based biosensors. Impedimetric biosensors detect affinity binding of target biomolecular structures such as antigens or DNA to a sensor surface as a result of the electric field between the electrodes changing due to the presence of the targeted biomolecule. As impedimetric sensing avoids the need of labelling the target, it is an attractive direct method of biosensing [32-34]. Nano-scaled electrodes detect events occurring on or in close proximity to the electrode surfaces. Scaling down the dimensions of electrochemical detectors offers new possibilities in terms of sensitivity and signal to background discrimination. Work will therefore have to concentrate on the further miniaturisation of the electrodes. However, as electrode areas decrease, so the interface impedances increase and the associated difficulties in accurate measurement. The key to success is in the choice of electrode and, in particular, the surface topography of the fabricated electrodes.

The immobilisation of biomolecules on the miniature sensors is also a key area of research and a range of analytical techniques have been used to study this facet of sensor fabrication – SPM, AES, XPS, CV, SIMS, EIS, IR/UV-vis spectroscopy. Published work indicates that it is the electrode-interface impedance which is the most sensitive to the immobilisation of biomolecules on the surface [34] and hence researchers should use a 3-electrode technique. Modelling and interpretation of EIS measurements will also enable the technique to approach its full potential.

5. Nanotechnology

Nanotechnology offers much promise for new sensor devices particularly in the biomedical sector. Miniaturisation, integration, nano-fabrication, quantum effects and the joining of disciplines such as biology, physics and engineering in particular offer many new opportunities for new scientific discoveries.

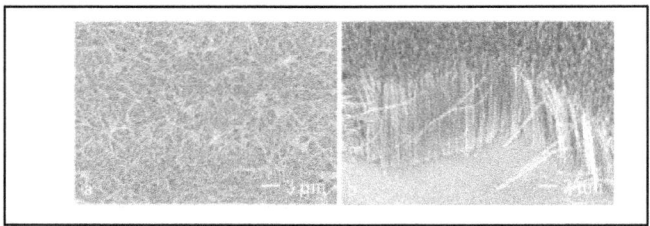

Figure 3. Nanotube forests suitable for biosensing electrodes.

Among the anticipated applications of carbon nanotubes (as shown in Figure 3), CNTs is their use as components in miniature biological devices such as probes and sensors. A nanotube might provide the finest needle for in vivo probing, for example monitoring chemical dynamics at the single cell level. These devices exhibit advantages over existing technology not only in size but also in performance. The better performance of the CNT electrodes in detecting biomolecules in solutions in comparison to the conventional used carbon electrodes lies in the high conductance of CNTs, which is suitable for the promotion of fast electron transfer, as well as in their inherent high surface area and tubular structure.

Several issues are important regarding CNT biosystems. One of them is development of chemical methods to immobilise biological molecules onto CNTs in a reliable manner. Central to tackling this issue is surface functionalisation of CNT and elucidating the interfaces and interactions between CNT and biosystems. Currently our overall understanding of the interactions between protein molecules and CNT surfaces is immature, in that we generally lack mechanistic and predictive structure reactivity relations. Projects seek to provide insights into the nature of the biomolecular junction and utilise that knowledge in the design of smart nanotubes that are bio-engineered and tailored–designed so as to accomplish detection of micro-organisms and biomolecules with high sensitivity and selectivity.

References

[1]   Misiano DR, Meyerhoff ME, Collinson ME. Current and future directions in the technology relating to bedside testing of critically ill patients. Chest 1990; 97: 204S-14S.
[2]   Ehrmeyer S, Burnett RW, Christiansen TF, Van Kessel AL, et al. Blood gas pre- analytical considerations: specimen collection, calibration, and controls. NCCLS Publication 27-A. Wayne, Pa: NCCLS, 1993; 13;6.
[3]   P Lemoine, P Mailley, M Hyland, J McLaughlin, E McAdams, J Anderson, A Lynch, D Diamond, M Leader Swelling and delamination of multi-electrode sensor arrays studied by variable-pressure scanning electron microscopy J Biomed Mater Res, 50, 313-321, 2000
[4]   D'Orazio PA, Maley TC, McCaffrey RR, Chan AC, et al. Planar (bio)sensors for critical care diagnosis. Clin Chem 1997; 43: 1804-05.
[5]   C. P. Price; Medical and Economic Outcomes of Point-of-Care Testing; Clinical Chemistry and Laboratory Medicine; 2002; 40; 3; 246-251.
[6]   J. Bennett, C. Cervantes, S Pachecho; Point-of-care testing: inspection preparedness; Perfusion 2000; 15; 137-142.
[7]   J. Khan, L.H. Saal, M.L. Bitner, et al; Expression profiling in cancer using cDNA microarrays; electrophoresis 1999; 20; 223-229.
[8]   L. DeFrancesco, MicroArrays in the New Millenium; part I; 2000; http://www.bioresearchonline.com
[9]   R.C. McGlennen; Miniaturization Technologies for Molecular Diagnostics; Clinical Chemistry 2001, 47:3, 393-402.
[10]   C. Henke; DNA chip technologies; part 3: What does the future hold?; 1999; http://www.devicelink.com/ivdt/archive/99/01/008.html
[11]   M.A. Schwarz, P.C. Hauser; Recent developments in detection methods for microfabricated analytical devices; Lab on a Chip; 2001; 1; 1-6.
[12]   Davis, T. M. and Wilson, W. D.; Determination of the Refractive Index Increments of Small Molecules for Correction of Surface Plasmon Resonance Data; Analytical Biochemistry ;284: 348-353; (10-9-2000).
[13]   Hall, D.; Use of Optical Biosensors for the Study of Mechanistically Concerted Surface Adsorption Processes; Analytical Biochemistry ;288: 109-125; (15-1-2001).
[14]   Kretschmann, E. and Reather, H.; Radiative decay of nonradiative surface plasmon excited by light.; Z.Naturf. ;23A: 2135-2136; (1968).
[15]   Markey, F.; What is SPR anyway?; Bia Journal ;1: 14-17; (1999).
[16]   Nagata, K. and Handa, H.; Rela-Time Analysis of Biomelecular Interactions; (2000).
[17]   Otto, A; A new method for exciting non-radioactive surface plasma oscillations.; Phys.Stat.Sol ;26: K99-K101; (1968).
[18]   Otto, A.; Exitation of nonradiative surface plasma waves in silver by the method of frustrated total reflection.; Z Phys ;216: 398-410; (1968).
[19]   Quinn, J. G. et all ; Development and application of surface plasmon resonance-based biosensors for the detection of cell-ligand interactions.; Analytical Biochemistry ;281: 135-143; (1-6-2000).
[20]   Baird, C. L. and Myszka, D. G.; Current and emerging commercial optical biosensors; J.Mol.Recognit. ;14: 261-268; (2001).
[21]   Ward, L. D. and Winzor, D. J.; Relative merits of optical biosensors based on flow-cell and cuvette designs; Analytical Biochemistry ;285: 179-193; (15-10-2000).
[22]   Weinberger, S. R. et all ; Recent trends in protein biochip technology; Pharmacogenomics. ;1: 395-416; (2000).
[23]   'Bioelectrical Impedance Techniques in Medicine', J-P. Morucci et al., Critical Reviews in Biomedical Engineering, 1996, vol.24, issues 4-6.

[24] Anthony Guiseppi-Elie, Ann M. Wilson, Thomas S. Oh, Andrew R. Sujdak, Ellen M. Davies, Sheldon P. Wesson, Gary E. Wnek, Philippe Lam, Gary C. Tepper, Oliver Bogler, Gary L. Bowlin, John Alexander and Robert J. Mattauch, "Microfabricated Impedimetric Array Chemical and Biological Sensors Using Smart Recognition-Transduction Electroconductive Hydrogels" NIST-ATP Workshop on Chemical Sensors and Biosensors, The Los Angeles Airport Hilton, Los Angeles, CA, USA, July 8 - 9, 1998.

[25] W. Laureyn, D. Nelis, P. Van Gerwen, K. Baert, L. Hermans, R. Magnée, J.-J. Pireaux; G. Maes, "Nanoscaled interdigitated titanium electrodes for impedimetric biosensing", Sensors and Actuators B, 68 (1-3) (2000) pp. 360-370].

[26] E.T. McAdams and J. Jossinet (1995) "Problems in equivalent circuit modelling of the electrical properties of biological tissues" Bioelectrochem & Bioenergetics, 40, 147 – 152.

[27] E.T. McAdams (1997) "Modelling the 'Constant Phase Angle' Behaviour: Potential Pitfalls" Invited talk. Solartron Seminar on 'Applications of Electrochemistry in Sensor Development', Department of Chemistry, University of Southampton, 11 February.

[28] E.T. McAdams, A. Lackermeier, J. A. McLaughlin and D. Macken. "The linear and non-linear electrical properties of the electrode-electrolyte interface.". Biosensors & Bioelectronics. 10, 67-74. 1995.

[29] J. Wegener, C.R. Keese, I. Giaever (2000) Electric cell-substrate impedance sensing as a non-invasive means to follow the kinetics of cell spreading on artificial surfaces. Exp. Cell Res., 259 158-166.

[30] J. Wegener, M. Sieber, H.-J. Galla (1996) Impedance analysis of epithelial and endothelial cell monolayers cultured on gold surfaces. J. Biochem. Biophys. Methods 32 151-170.

[31] Schmukler, R. 1999. Mammalian gene transfer by low voltage electroporation. Bioelectromagnetics Society's Therapeutic Benefits of Electromagnetic Fields Workshop. February. Washington, USA.

[32] Van Gerwen, P., Laureyn, W., Laureys, W., Huyberechts, G., Op De Beeck, M., Baert, K., Suls, J., Sansen, W., Jacobs, P., Hermans, L., Mertens, R. (1998) Nanoscaled interdigitated electrode arrays for biochemical sensors. Sensors and Actuators B, 49, 73-80.

[33] Laureyn, W., Nelis, D., Van Gerwen, P., Baert, K., Hermans, L. and Macs, G. (1999) Nanoscaled Interdigitated Titanium Electrodes for Impedimetric Biosensing. Eurosensors XIII, Micro Analysis Systems, 347-350.

[34] Laureyn, W. Nelis, D. Van Gerwen, P., Baert, K., Hermans, L., Magneee, R., Pireaux, J.J., Maes, G. (2000) Nanoscaled interdigitated titanium electrodes for impedimetric biosensing. Sensors and Actuators B-Chemical, 360-370.

Personalised Health Management Systems
C.D. Nugent et al. (Eds.)
IOS Press, 2005

Bioimpedance and p-Health

Jacques JOSSINET[1]

Institut National de la Santé et de la Recherche Médicale (INSERM)
INSERM U556, Lyon, France

Abstract. Bio-impedance is the electrical impedance of living matter. Bio-impedance methods present a range of known advantages for medical and clinical applications including low-cost, non-invasiveness and harmlessness. The measured parameter reflects the physiological and pathological processes that take place within human body. The technological progress in instrumentation has significantly contributed to the progress that has been observed during the last past decades in impedance spectroscopy and electrical impedance tomography. Although bioimpedance is not a physiological parameter, the method enables tissue characterisation and functional monitoring and can contribute to the monitoring of the health status of a person. The association of this flexible and versatile method with micro-electronics and wireless telecommunication systems opens a new field of potential applications.

Keywords. Electrical bioimpedance, impedance spectroscopy, plethysmography, electrical impedance tomography, tissue characterisation, monitoring.

Introduction

Bioimpedance is by definition the electrical impedance of living substance, namely the human body in the context of p-health. The engineer's definition of electrical impedance is the complex ratio of sinusoidal voltage to current across a circuit element. The term bioimpedance also applies to measurement carried out on samples ex vivo such as biopsies, excised tissue samples, blood samples, body fluids, suspensions of cells, cell broths and cultured cells. The conduction observed at the macroscopic level results from the microscopic structure of the medium [1,2]. The understanding of the relationship between a tissue's structure and its electric and dielectric properties has improved concomitantly with the knowledge progressively gained in cell biophysics and the technological progress in instrumentation and data processing techniques [3]. The major impedance methods for biomedical application are impedance spectroscopy, impedance plethysmography and

---

[1] Corresponding Author: INSERM U556, 151 Cours Albert Thomas, 69424 Lyon cedex 03, France; E-mail:jossinet@lyon.inserm.fr.

impedance imaging. Their features are described in the following sections with particular attention to the requirements and operation conditions of personalised health systems.

Over the last past decades, the research in bioimpedance has received significant support from the European Commission. For instance, bioimpedance methods were included in the workshop on "*Bioelectric and Thermal Sensors*" held in Lyon, 1991 as part of the European programme "*University-Enterprise Training Partnership*", UETP/COMETT-BME [4]. The emergence of Electrical Impedance Tomography was supported by the COMAC-BME in the eighties and nineties. After the workshops in Sheffield, 1986 and Lyon, 1987, the two consecutive Concerted Actions on Electrical Impedance Imaging gave rise to active cooperation between a rapidly growing number of European teams and resulted in the existing European leadership this field [5,6,7,8].

1. Electric and Dielectric Properties of Tissue

The human body is obviously not an electrical circuit; it is a heterogeneous, anisotropic, deformable volume conductor. The presence of cells gives cellular media unique electric and dielectric properties [9,10]. In the frequency range used for impedance measurement, the active biological properties of the cell membrane do not play a significant role. The influence of the cell membrane can be described in terms of membrane passive conductance (nearly zero in most cases) and capacitance. The latter results from the capacitor-like structure formed by the cell membrane, the interstitial space and the intracellular space (endoplasm).

It has long been observed that living tissue, and more generally biological substances, differs from "pure conductors" and "pure capacitors" [11,12]. Biological media are characterised at the macroscopic level either by their "complex conductivity", termed "admittivity" and usually denoted σ^*, or by their "complex dielectric permittivity", generally denoted ε^*. These quantities are not independent, as both must account for the electric and dielectric properties of the medium. In Eq. (1), "j" is the base of imaginary numbers, ω is the angular frequency and ε_0 is the dielectric permittivity of a vacuum:

$$\sigma^* = j\omega\varepsilon_0\varepsilon^* \qquad\qquad\qquad (1)$$

The electric DC conductivities of the interstitial space and endoplasm are practically constant in the frequency range used for impedance measurement. In this frequency range, several types of dielectric phenomena can take place within the medium. Consequently, σ^* and ε^* vary with the applied signal frequency giving rise to three principal types of dispersion. The α-dispersion occurs near the cell surface at very low frequency. The β-dispersion is due to the accumulation of charges at interfaces at radio-frequencies (Maxwell-Wagner structural relaxation). The γ-dispersion is due to the orientation of polar molecules (water) at very high frequencies. The archetypal admittivity function against frequency in a tissue with a single dispersion is given by Eq.(2):

$$\sigma^* = \sigma_\infty + (\sigma_0 - \sigma_\infty)/\left(1 + (jf/f_0)^m\right) \tag{2}$$

In the complex plane (resistance, capacitance) the plot of this equation is a circular arc, the centre of which is shifted below the real axis. The intercepts of the arc with this axis are the low frequency limit conductance σ_0 and the high frequency limit conductance, σ_∞. The former is the admittance of the interstitial space, while the latter is predominantly due to the intracellular medium. The values of the fractional power, m, and characteristic frequency, f_0, depend on the parameters of the cells, including shape, concentration, orientation and cell membrane response.

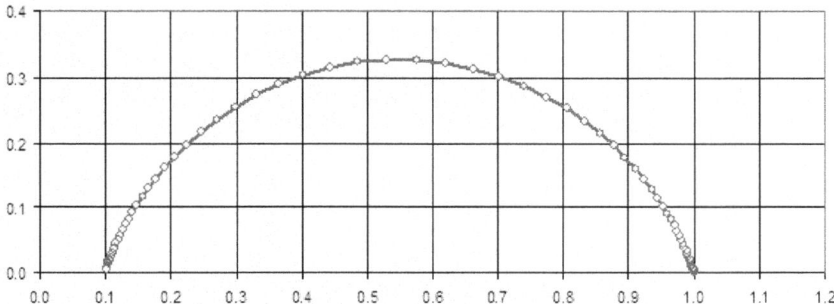

Figure 1. Example of a circular arc calculated using realistic values. Units are S/m on both axes ($\sigma_0 = 1$ S/m, $\sigma_\infty = 0.1$ S/m, m = 0.8, $f_0 = 10$ kHz). The reduction of experimental points to a small set of parameters enables the comparison between impedance data obtained at different frequencies.

Fitting a circular arc to the experiment points enables the calculation of the above four parameters. The response of a tissue obeying the above equation may be described by an equivalent circuit model consisting of two resistances and a pseudo-capacitance [2,13]. The detailed review of such models is beyond the scope of this paper.

2. Impedance Methods

The key point of bioimpedance measurement is that the structure of a tissue at the cellular level determines the observed macroscopic impedance. The physiological and pathological processes that can take place within a tissue affect the cellular structure and consequently produce impedance changes. For this reason, bioimpedance enables both tissue characterisation and functional monitoring

2.1. Impedance Spectroscopy

Impedance spectroscopy is the study of a tissue's impedance within a given frequency range for tissue characterisation. The purpose of this type of measurement is to gain physiological and pathological information about the examined tissue [14,15]. The interpretation of data is a two-step process. The first step constitutes the estimation of σ_0 and ε_0 from the measured impedance values. The second step is the extraction of the physiological information from the observed values or changes in their values.

2.2. Impedance Plethysmography

This method consists of the determination of periodic volume changes in bodily parts by recording an impedance signal which can be related to, for example, cardiac activity or blood flow. This method was studied to provide a system capable of measuring cardiac output in the first astronauts and was termed "impedocardiography". The basic principle is the so-called "parallel conductor model" [16,17,18]. Although it appeared subject to errors due to the variability in human anatomy, this method remains useful in monitoring cardiac function in situations where the patient acts as his (her) own reference. Signal processing enables the calculation of several indices relating to heart performance, including the contractility index.

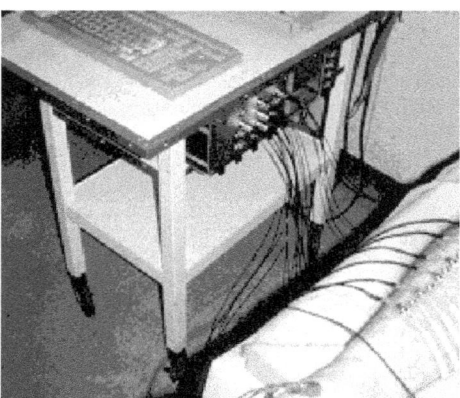

Figure 2. Measurement of pulse wave velocity in normal subjects and diabetic patients using a multi-channel impedance device and an array of screen-printed electrodes (technology developed at the Northern Ireland Bio-Engineering Centre, University of Ulster).

In limbs, this method has given rise to venous occlusion plethysmography, the study of blood flow and the measurement of pulse wave velocity for the characterisation of arterial wall stiffness [19]. Respiratory function can also be monitored using thoracic impedance measurement. It is crucial in this case to minimise the influence of motion artefact.

2.3. Impedance Imaging

Impedance imaging is based on multiple impedance measurements. The parameter of interest is the electric conductivity inside the body. The collected data consist either of values of transimpedance used for 2D mapping (thorax mapping, breast imaging, skin mapping) or tomographic data obtained by multiplexing a set of electrodes and processed by appropriate image reconstruction algorithms. This modality is termed Electrical Impedance Tomography (EIT) [7,8]. The usual implementation of EIT consists of electrodes located at the circumference of a cross-section of the body. EIT reconstruction algorithms consist of the resolution of the inverse problem associated to the second order equation: $\nabla.\nabla(\sigma V)=0$. This problem is inherently ill-posed because the sensitivity of surface electrodes decreases strongly from the surface to the deep regions of the body. The contribution of internal regions to the measured signal is low and sensitive to noise. The boundary conditions needed to solve the inverse problem are the object shape, the applied signals and the measured signals. Due to the nature of the governing equation, impedance imaging has relatively low spatial resolution compared to the other imaging techniques. On the other hand, Electrical Impedance Tomography presents high time-resolution and is highly sensitive to small conductivity changes inside the body, even though it cannot determine accurately their location. Impedance imaging gives rise to several modalities such as Electrical Impedance Endotomography where the electrodes are located on a probe placed at the centre of the region of interest for local measurements [20,21].

3. What Bioimpedance Can Tell Us

The information extracted from impedance values depends on the method used for data collection. As skin is an insulating barrier, conductive electrodes must be used. The design of electrode systems not only ensure the quality of contact between body and instrumentation, but also permits the optimisation of the volume explored. The appropriate design and placement of an electrode enable the fitting of the sensitivity domain of the sensor to the desired region of interest. Table I shows examples of practical applications of impedance measurement. BIA (bioimpedance analysis) is the name given to the study of body composition, including the determination of total body water and fat free mass.

Table I. Examples of operating conditions and associated information.

whole body	single frequency, BIA, multiple frequency	body composition, body water
segmental measurements	single frequency, multiple frequency	body composition, fat free mass, fluid shifts
thorax, abdomen	functional monitoring	heart function, respiration gastric emptying
limbs	impedance plethysmography	bloodflow, pulse wave velocity
local measurements	impedance spectroscopy,	detection of oedema,

	tissue characterisation,	inflammation, malignancy
skin and subcutaneous tissue characterisation	impedance spectroscopy impedance mapping	skin diseases, monitoring of burns and wound healing
local measurements	impedance spectroscopy, tissue characterisation,	detection of oedema, inflammation,malignancy
thorax, abdomen, skull, limbs, breast	Impedance tomography single or multiple frequency	dynamic imaging, real time imaging, tissue characterisation

4. Bioimpedance in p-Health?

Bioimpedance methods are usable and have been used in a wide field of applications relating to health in hospitals, medical centres and at general practitioners' clinics. The study of body composition has given rise to numerous studies in nutrition and sport. The low cost and non-invasiveness are appropriate for disease prevention and screening. The user-friendliness is conducive to integration in homecare systems. The flexibility of bioimpedance impedance methods makes it easy to incorporate this type of measurement into a wide range of applications.

The history of bio-impedance and the present technological progress indicates possible future applications. The association of impedance to main frame computers improved the signal processing even if the measurements had to be carried out in the computer room. More recently, microcomputers enabled the design of impedance systems for patient's bedside. Presently, many impedance systems consist of handheld devices. It can therefore be expected that miniaturised impedance modules can be associated with or incorporated into portable/wearable systems and intelligent apparel. However, for ambulatory applications, the basic features of bioimpedance methods should not be ignored at the stage of system specification. The following section summarises the known advantages and drawbacks of impedance methods for the evaluation of their compatibility with the requirements of p-health.

4.1. Pros and Cons of Bioimpedance Methods

4.1.1. Advantages

Low cost
Non-invasiveness or minimal invasiveness (oesophageal gastric probes, urethral probes)
Harmlessness for the patient and the operator
Low power consumption
Miniaturisation possible for portable or wearable devices
Electrode technology available

4.1.2. Drawbacks

Impedance is not a physiological parameter, although it reflects biological processes
Multiple factors of influence (tissue structure, anisotropy, temperature, motion)
Inherently limited spatial resolution
Signal recording generally needs subject's cooperation

5. Conclusion

The physical bases of impedance measurement have been well established. Consequently, the incorporation of impedance measurement in p-health systems should not require excessive fundamental research, so that the effort could focus on technical implementation. The success of a final application requires at least two crucial conditions: the accurate definition of the information desired and the operational conditions to collect it. The above pros and cons may serve as guidelines for the integration of bioimpedance in p-health applications. Furthermore, the emergence of micro-technology opens new prospects for the bioimpedance method. In particular, impedance measurement at the cellular level enables recording of cell activity, such as cellular growth and tumour development.

References

[1]   H.P. Schwan, Analysis of dielectric data : Experience gained with biological material, *IEEE Trans.*, EI-**20**(6) (1985), 913-922.
[2]   K.R. Foster and H.P. Schwan, Dielectric properties of tissues and biological materials: a critical review, *CRC Critical Reviews in Biomedical Engineering*, **17**(1) (1989), 25-104.
[3]   H.P. Schwan and S. Takashima, Electrical conduction and dielectric behavior in biological systems, *Encyclopedia of Applied Physics*, VCH Publishers Inc., **5** (1993), 177-200.
[4]   A. Dittmar, J. Jossinet, E.T. McAdams *et al.*, Proc. UETP/COMETT-BME seminar on Medical Bioelectric and Thermal Surface Sensors, 26-28 June, Lyon, *Innov. Techn. Biol. Med.*, Special Issue, **12**(1) (1991).
[5]   B.H. Brown, D.C. Barber and L. Tarassenko, Proc. 1st European workshop "Electrical impedance Tomography – Applied potential tomography, 2-4 July, Sheffield, UK, Comac-BME, *Clin. Phys. and Physiol. Meas.*, Special Issue , **8**(Suppl. A) (1987).
[6]   B.H. Brown, D.C. Barber and J. Jossinet, Proc. 2nd European workshop on Electrical impedance Tomography – Applied potential tomography, 21-23 Oct1987, Lyon, France, Comac-BME, *Clin. Phys. and Physiol. Meas.*, Special Issue, **9**(Suppl. A) (1988).
[7]   K. Boone, D. Barber and B.H. Brown, Imaging with electricity: report of the European concerted action on impedance tomography, *J. Med.Eng. Technol.*, **21**(6) (1997), 201-232.
[8]   A.M. Dijkstra, B.H. Brown *et al.*, Clinical applications of electrical impedance tomography, *J. Med. Eng. Technol.*, **17**(3) (1993), 89-98.
[9]   L. Geddes and L.E. Baker, The specific resistance of biological material- A compendium of data for the biomedical engineer and physiologist, *Med. Biol. Eng.*, **5** (1967), 271-93.
[10] R.D. Stoy, K.R. Foster and H.P. Schwan, Dielectric properties of mammalian tissues from 0.1 to 100 MHz:A summary of recent data, *Phys. Med. Biol.*, **27** (1982), 501-513.
[11] E.T. McAdams and J. Jossinet, Epidermial/tissue impedance: an historical overview, *Phys. Meas.*, **16**(Suppl. 3A) (1995), A1-A14.
[12] J. Jossinet, Proc. CAIT workshop on the modeling of cellular media in electrical Impedance Tomography, 9-10 June 1995, Lyon, France, *Innov. Techn. Biol. Med.*, Thematic Issue, **16**(6) (1995).

[13] E.T. McAdams and J. Jossinet, Problems in equivalent circuit modelling of the electrical properties of biological tissues, *Bioelectrochemistry and Bioenergetics*, **40** (1996), 147-152.

[14] J. Jossinet *et al.*, Quantitative technique for bio-electrical spectroscopy, *J. Biomed. Eng.*, **7** (1985), 289-294.

[15] J. Jossinet, The impedivity of freshly excised human breast tissue, *Physiol. Meas.*, **19** (1998), 61-75.

[16] J. Nyboer, Electrical impedance plethysmography: A physical and physiologic approach to peripheral vascular study, *Circ.*, **2** (1950), 811-821.

[17] W.G. Kubicek, R.P. Patterson and D.A. Witsoe, Impedance cardiography as a noninvasive method of monitoring cardiac function and other parameters of the cardiovascular system, *Ann. NY Acad. Sci*, **170** (1970), 724-732.

[18] J. Jossinet, G. Leftheriotis *et al.*, A computerized bio-electrical cardiac monitor, *Computers in Medicine and Biology*, **20**(4) (1990), 253-260.

[19] F. Risacher, J. Jossinet, E.T. McAdams *et al.*, Impedance plethysmography for the evaluation of pulse wave velocity in limbs, *Biomed. Eng. and Comput.*, **31** (1993), 318-322.

[20] J. Jossinet, E. Marry, A. Montalibet *et al.*, Electrical Impedance Endo-Tomography: Imaging tissue from inside", *IEEE Trans. on Medical Imaging*, **21**(6) (2002), 560-565.

[21] J. Jossinet, E. Marry and A. Matias, Electrical Impedance Endotomography, *Physics in Medecine and Biology*, **47**(13) (2002), 2189-2202.

Personalised Health Management Systems
C.D. Nugent et al. (Eds.)
IOS Press, 2005

Vital Sign Monitoring for Elderly at Home: Development of a Compound Sensor for Pulse Rate and Motion

K.W. SUM [a, b], Y.P. ZHENG [a 1], and A. F. T. MAK [a]

[a] Rehabilitation Engineering Center, Hong Kong Polytechnic University, Hong Kong
[b] Department of EEE, The University of Hong Kong, Hong Kong

Abstract. This paper describes the development of a miniaturized wearable vital sign monitor which is aimed for use by elderly at home. The development of a compound sensor for pulse rate, motion, and skin temperature is reported. A pair of infrared sensor working in reflection mode was used to detect the pulse rate from various sites over the body including the wrist and finger. Meanwhile, a motion sensor was used to detect the motion of the body. In addition, the temperature on the skin surface was sensed by a semiconductor temperature sensor. A prototype has been built into a box with a dimension of 2 x 2.5 x 4 cm^3. The device includes the sensors, microprocessor, circuits, battery, and a wireless transceiver for communicating data with a data terminal.

Keywords. Vital Sign Monitoring, Elderly Healthcare, e-Healthcare, Wearable Device, Compound Sensor, Biomedical Engineering.

Introduction

There is an increasing need for the vital sign monitoring when a subject is at home, particularly for an elderly person at home alone. According to a recent government statistics, there are currently more than 1 million of the total Hong Kong population (7 million) aged over 60, whilst 800,000 of them aged over 65. The number should be able to reflect the global situation. A related concern is the sharp increase of "old old", i.e. those aged over 80 or above. The safety of the vulnerable including the elderly and the disabled when they need to stay home by themselves is a big social concern. This concern continues to grow as the overall population ages, and as the economic situation requires parents and other adults of the family all to work longer hours. Many recent research and development projects have been targeted on health care monitoring devices [1-3]. According to different applications, they were focused on different technology aspects to optimize their solutions. The overall aim of this project is to develop a vital sign monitoring system for elderly at home. In this chapter, the

---

[1] Corresponding author: Dr. Y.P. Zheng, Rehabilitation Engineering Center, Hong Kong Polytechnic University, Hong Kong; Email: ypzheng@ieee.org.

development of a compound sensor for pulse rate and motion is reported. A pair of infrared sensors working in reflection mode was used to detect the pulse rate from various sites over the body including the wrist and finger. Meanwhile, a motion sensor was used to detect the motion of the body. In addition, the temperature on the skin surface was sensed by a semiconductor temperature sensor. A prototype has been build into a box with a dimension of 2 x 2.5 x 4 cm^3. The device includes the sensors, microprocessor, circuits, battery, and a wireless transceiver for communicating data with a station.

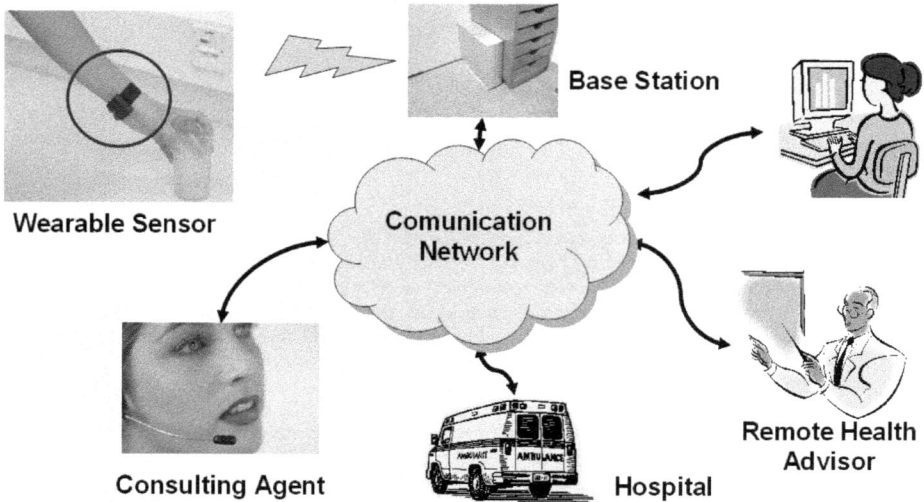

Figure 1. Overall diagram of the wearable vital sign sensor together with its base station and the alarm system. Different parties could be notified when an abnormal patterns of vital signs were detected by the base station.

1. System Design Overview

The major goal of this project was to develop a wearable vital sign monitor for elderly. Since the elderly might not be capable to interact with new technologies and might not be willing to use complex devices in a continuously way, many design considerations had to be addressed for a multi-sensor integrated monitoring device.

One of the most important considerations was that the device should be easy to operate. The user group of our application was in the age of over 60. Most of them were living alone and were using the device by themselves. Therefore, sophisticated sensor wiring or any other complex operating procedures had to be avoided. Our device was fabricated in different shapes, so that it could be used on different portion of the human body. The prototype was built as a wrist-watch. The design idea was that by using an unobtrusive wrist-worn device, monitoring could be performed without interfering with the subjects' everyday activities and without restricting their mobility. All of the sensing methods were non-invasive to avoid any discomfort to the subject.

The vital sign signals collected by the wearable sensor were be analyzed by a base station, which would send alarm signals to the concerned parties when an abnormal pattern of the vital signs were detected. Figure 1 shows the overall diagram of how the alarm system worked. The base station could automatically send alarms via a telephone line, Internet, or other communication networks according to the preset telephone numbers and other address information.

The power consumption of device is a key consideration. The vital sign monitor was used by the elderly continuously at home. It is not feasible to replace or recharge the battery everyday as this would reduce the willingness of the elderly to use the device. The size of the device was also important for wearable devices. A bulky design would not be feasible for practical applications. Figure 2 shows the functional block diagram of the wearable device. Details of the sensors and methodology are described in the following sections.

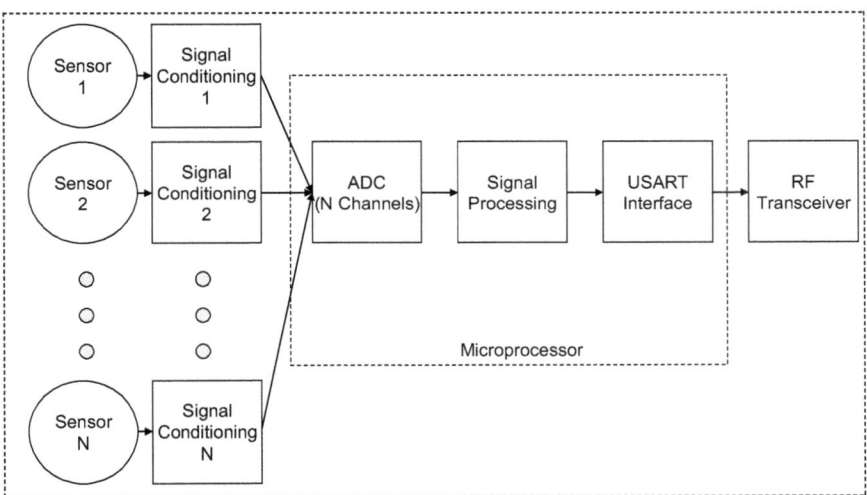

Figure 2. Functional block diagram of the wearable device. The microprocessor was used to digitize the vital sign signals and to control the transmission of the data to the based station.

2. Sensors

The sensors are the major interfaces between the wearable device and the human body. Three different sensors were integrated in the current compound vital sign sensor. They were used to sense non-invasively the heart pulse, body motion and skin temperature.

2.1. Pulse Sensor

The photoplethysmography (PPG) technique was used to sense the heart pulse non-invasively. This technique makes use of visible or invisible light on a small area of the human body in order to detect the variation of the blood flow volume. In our design, an infrared light emitter and detector was used to capture the variation of the reflected light by the body surface. During systole, the blood volume increases; during diastole, it decreases. The PPG output reflects changes in blood volume in the peripheral circulation.

There are two major types of PPG. One is performed using penetration and the other is using reflection. The peak wavelengths of the infrared emitter and detector pairs are normally in the range of 690nm to 940nm. If the infrared light has a smaller peak wavelength, the frequency of the emitted infrared light will be higher. Hence, the penetration capability of the infrared light will be increased. Therefore, the peak wavelengths of the infrared sensors have to be carefully selected for different sensing methods.

In our design, we used the reflective sensing method. The wavelength of the infrared sensor was around 900 nm to optimize the measurement. There were two major advantages of choosing reflective mode. Firstly, this reduced the power consumption which wasted through penetration to the back of the body tissue. Secondly, this allowed the sensor to be used on various parts of the body since the penetration mode cannot be applied, for example, at the wrist and the neck.

The captured signal was then passed through a second ordered low pass filter and amplifier to improve the signal condition to a level where was acceptable by the microprocessor for digitization and subsequent heart rate calculation.

2.2. Motion Sensor

The motion sensor was used to measure the body movement of the subject. There were two major functions for integrating a motion sensor into the device. Firstly, most of the elderly might have difficulty in movement and most accidents happened at home, caused by falls. Monitoring the movement of the subject could help to determine whether the subject fell or not. If the subject fell, immediate help might be required. Secondly, since there might have motion artifacts in the measured signals from other sensors, this motion information was useful to act as a reference signal to minimize the motion artifact.

We used the accelerometer as the motion sensor. The Analog Device ADXL311 is a low cost, low power, complete dual-axis accelerometer with signal conditioned voltage outputs all on a single monolithic IC. The accelerometer measures the acceleration with a full-scale range of $\pm 2g$ and can measure both dynamic acceleration (e.g. vibration) and static acceleration (e.g. gravity). The outputs were analog voltages proportional to the acceleration. In our application, the absolute magnitude of the output voltage was not important. Instead, we were interested in the relative variations which showed the relative motion of the body. In addition, this accelerometer was available in a very compact package as small as a 5 x 5 x 2mm^3 8-terminal hermetic ceramic leadless chip carrier (CLCC) package. This facilitated the miniaturization of our devices.

2.3. Temperature Sensor

In our device, we were incorporating different sensors for different vital sign detection and monitoring. One of the obvious vital signs was the body temperature. Since this was a non-invasive monitoring device, only the skin temperature was considered. We used the National Semiconductor LM35 precision centigrade temperature sensor. LM35 is a precision integrated-circuit temperature sensor, whose output voltage is linearly proportional to the Celsius (Centigrade) temperature. LM35 does not require any external calibration or trimming and provides typical accuracies of ±0.25°C at room temperature and ±0.75°C over a full -55 to +150°C temperature range. This reduced the number of extra components of the circuit. Low cost was assured by trimming and calibration at the wafer level. LM35's low output impedance, linear output, and precise inherent calibration make interfacing to readout or control circuitry especially easy. LM35 is small in size with TO-92 plastic package.

3. Microprocessor

The microprocessor was the heart of the whole wearable device. It performed several key functions including analog-to-digital (A/D) conversion, signal processing, and serial communication interface. We used an Microchip PIC18F series microprocessor, which was an enhanced FLASH microcontroller with 10-bit A/D and nano-watt technology. There were maximum 7 A/D converters which allowed conversion of the analog input signals to the corresponding 10-bit digital numbers. After digitizing the analog voltage from different sensors, the data was post processed to ensure the integrity of the input data.   Also, the heart rate of subject could be calculated in the microprocessor or at the remote terminal. In addition, the microprocessor includes a universal synchronous asynchronous receiver transmitter (USART) module. The USART was configured to communicate with the radio frequency transmitter IC in our wearable device.

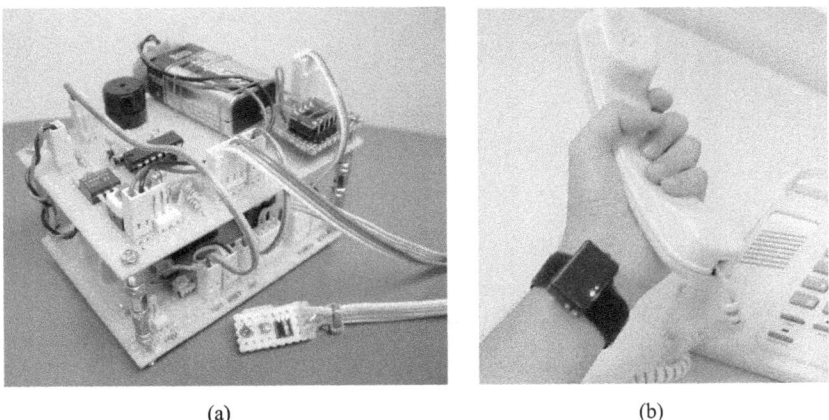

(a)   (b)

Figure 3. The prototypes of the vital sign sensors. (a) The initial testing board; and (b) the miniaturized prototypes with a dimension of 2 x 2.5 x 4 cm^3, which could be worn on the wrist of the subject.

4. Wireless Communication

The wireless communication provided an interface between the monitoring device and the data terminal. The data terminal was expected to be installed inside the home of the subject. Therefore, the range of the air interface was limited in an area with a radius of less than 300 feet. We used a low-cost, ultra-low power consumption, and compact surface mount packaged radio frequency (RF) module from LINX. The transceiver accepted CMOS/TTL level data input which could be supplied with the USART output directly from the microprocessor. During standby or the input of a logic low, the carrier is fully suppressed and the transmitter consumes less than 2μA of current.

Figure 3 shows the vital sign measurement devices before and after miniaturization. Surface mounting components were used to reduce the required dimension for the circuit. A battery was also included in the wearable device shown in Figure 3b.

5. Data Terminal

The data terminal, i.e. the base station, was basically a desktop computer equipped with a RF transceiver and was installed with the system software. The data terminal received, stored, and processed all the vital sign data from the wearable monitor. The user interface of the system software is shown in Figure 4. It shows the waveforms of the heart pulses, skin temperature variations, and motion signal. In addition, it computed and displayed the pulse rate of the heart pulse. The data terminal sends alarm messages to the concerned parties using different communication networks when an abnormal pattern of the vital signs was detected.

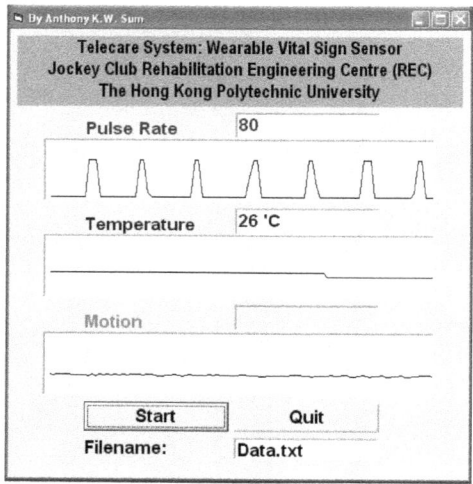

Figure 4. The user interface of the system software showing the pulse rate, skin temperature and motion activities. All the vital sign data could be recorded and the abnormal pattern being monitored in real-time.

6. Preliminary Results

The wearable monitor shown in Figure 3b has been successfully used to collected pulse, motion and skin temperature when it was worn at different locations including the wrist and fingers. The vital sign data could be successfully transmitted from the wearable monitor to the base station. Further improvements are being made to reduce its dimension and to increase the battery life. In addition, we noted that the pulse detection was sensitive to the pressure applied on the skin. A systematic study is being conducted to find the optimized pressure required for the pulse measurement. We also noted that motion artifacts could not be avoided when the wearable vital sign monitor was moved by the subject. Figure 5 shows three typical waveforms of the pulse and motion collected by monitor under the conditions of no motion, mild motion and strong motion, respectively. It could be observed that the artifacts in the pulse signals were highly correlated with the motion signals. We proposed a motion compensation method to reduce the influence of the motion artifacts to the pulse detection [4].

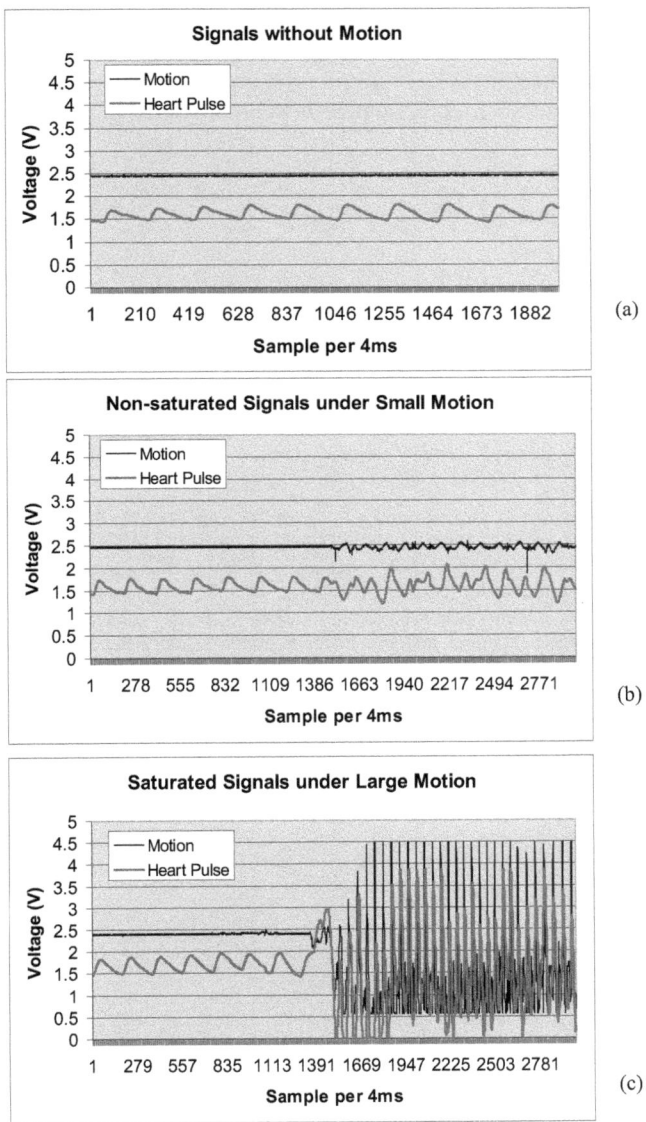

Figure 5. Typical waveforms of pulse and motion collected from a figure tip under different conditions of the hand. (a) No motion; (b) small motion; and (c) large motion.

7. Discussions and Conclusions

In this chapter, we introduced the development of a compound sensor for vital sign monitoring. The device could be used to monitor the heart rate, motion, and the skin temperature of the elderly at home. All the sensing technologies employed are non-invasive. The prototype of the device was compact with a dimension of 2 x 2.5 x 4 cm^3. Preliminary tests for the wearable sensor demonstrated that it was reliable in the collection of vital signs from different locations of the body. The detected motion signal was beneficial not only for the fall detection of the subject but also for the compensation of the motion artifacts to the other measured vital signs. More sensors are being integrated into the current prototype to enhance the functions for other potential vital signs, such as blood pressure and blood oxygen level.

Acknowledgements

The project was supported by a research fund from Hong Kong Jockey Club Charity. The authors would like to thanks all the team members of the Telecare project for their useful comments.

References

[1] U. Anliker, J.A. Ward, P. Lukowicz, G. Troster, F. Dolveck, M. Baer, F. Keita, E.B. Schenker, F. Catarsi, L. Coluccini, A. Belardinelli, D. Shklarski, M. Alon, E. Hirt, R. Schmid, and M. Vuskovic, "AMON: A wearable multiparameter medical monitoring and alert system", IEEE Transactions on Information in Biomedicine 8 (2004), 415-427.
[2] J. Bai, Y.H. Zhang, D.L. Shen, L.F. Wen, C.X. Ding, Z.J. Cui, F.H. Tian, B. Yu, B. Dai, and J.P. Zhang, "A portable ecg and blood pressure telemonitoring system", IEEE Engineering in Medicine and Biology 46 (1999), 63-70
[3] K. Doughty, K. Cameron, and P. Garner, "Three generations of telecare of the elderly", Journal of Telemedicine and Telecare 2 (1996), 71-80
[4] Y.P. Zheng, K.W. Sum, and A.F.T. Mak, "Portable motion compensated health monitoring device and its motion compensation scheme", State Intellectual Property Office of the People's Republic of China, Application No. 200410056044.2.

Personalised Health Management Systems
C.D. Nugent et al. (Eds.)
IOS Press, 2005

MyHeart: Fighting Cardio-Vascular Diseases by Preventive Lifestyle and Early Diagnosis

Ralf SCHMIDT, Josef LAUTER
Philips Research Laboratories, Germany

Abstract. Cardio-vascular diseases (CVD) are the leading cause of death. The MyHeart Project aims at empowering the citizens to fight cardio-vascular diseases by preventive lifestyle and early diagnosis. The main technical challenges in this project are the combination of novel wearable technologies (novel textile and electronic sensors, personalised algorithms, on-body computing) and user feedback and motivation concepts, in order to make a breakthrough towards new applications for prevention and early diagnose possible.

Keywords. Cardio-vascular diseases, textiles, prevention, personal healthcare.

Introduction

Cardio-vascular diseases (CVD) are the leading cause of death. In Europe over 20% of all citizens suffer from a chronic CVD and 45% of all deaths are due to CVD. Europe spends annually hundreds of billion Euros on CVD. The increasing aging of the population is a challenge for Europe to deliver its citizens healthcare at affordable costs. It is commonly accepted, that a healthy and preventive lifestyle as well as early diagnosis could systematically reduce the modifiable risk factors of CVD and save millions of live-years. The MyHeart mission is to empower the citizen to fight cardio-vascular diseases by preventive lifestyle and early diagnosis.

The starting point is to gain knowledge on a citizen's actual health status. Continuous monitoring of vital signs is mandatory for that. The approach is to integrate system solutions into functional clothes with integrated textile sensors. That is the definition of intelligent biomedical clothes. The processing consists of making diagnoses, detecting trends and react on it. Together with feedback devices that are able to interact with the user as well as with professional services this completes the MyHeart system.

This system supports citizens to fight modifiable CVD risk factors, helps to avoid acute events by personalized guidelines and feedback and motivates to maintain a healthy lifestyle. Objectives of MyHeart are to open up a new mass market for the European industry and to help to prevent CVD while reducing the overall EU healthcare costs. The consortium consists of 33 partners from 11 countries.

1. Project Objectives

1.1. Background - Mortality and morbidity of Cardio-Vascular Diseases

Cardio-vascular diseases (CVD) are the leading cause of death in developed countries. Roughly 45% of all deaths in the EU are due to CVD (Figure 1). More than 20% of all European citizens suffer from chronic CVDs. This disease class includes myocardial infarction, congestive heart failure, arrhythmias and stroke. Hypertension, high cholesterol, diabetes, stress and obesity are the main risk factors for developing CVD.

Having a high risk often means to suffer from limitations in daily life. Obese patients have severe limitation in their ability to follow an active lifestyle. After a major cardio-vascular event patients' quality of life is severely impaired.

Studies showed that 20 % of all myocardial infarction patients will develop depressions. The majority of patients live in such anxiety, that their ability to take actively part in social and economic life is limited.

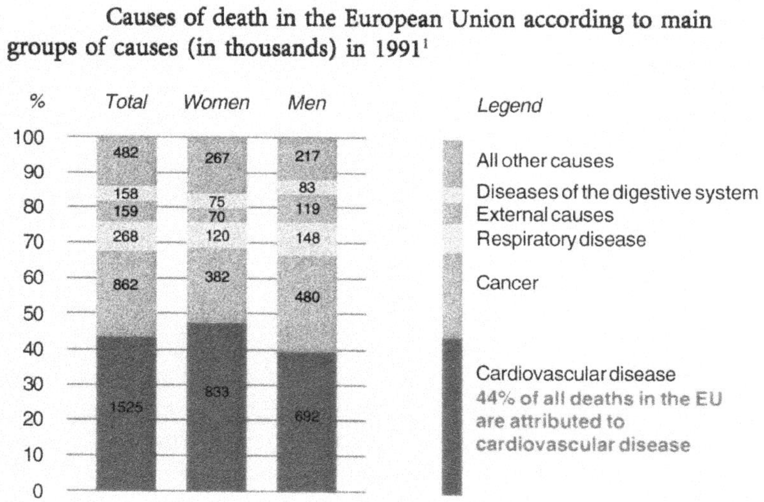

Figure 1. Mortality due to cardio-vascular and other diseases in the European Union. Source: Physical Activity and CVD prevention in the EU.

1.2. Healthcare expenditures in Europe for cardio-vascular diseases

CVD is not only a major threat in terms of mortality, morbidity and quality of life; it is also a major economic burden to all European countries. Annually Europe spends several hundred billion Euros on the management of CVD. The direct medical costs represent only one third of the overall cost for society. The major costs are the indirect costs to the community such as lost of productivity due to illness and premature death. In the USA cardio-vascular diseases account for a total of 329 billion dollars. In Germany 13% of all direct healthcare costs are due to CVD. The aging population in Europe will further increase the number of chronic CVD patients.

1.3. Preventive lifestyle and early diagnosis of CVD

The individual lifestyle is most important in reducing the modifiable risks for CVD. Cardiology societies have developed recommendations on the prevention of CVD diseases, improvement of the clinical outcome and the limitation of the recurrence of acute events after a first major event.

A healthy and preventive lifestyle as well as early diagnosis of heart diseases could save millions of life years each year and could significantly reduce the morbidity and improve the quality of life. Prevention systematically reduces the risk factors of cardio-vascular diseases and improves the medical outcome after an event.

Prevention and healthy lifestyle is a lifelong continuous process that cannot effectively be provided by the classical institutional points of care: hospitals, clinics and office based physicians. Although these institutions have the required concepts and expertise they are not capable to bring them to the citizen at home. These classical institutions offer only intermittent, episodically treatment, while prevention asks for a lifelong continuous change of habits and therefore for a continuous health-care delivery process. Novel methods are needed that provide continuous and ubiquitous access to medical excellence in a cost-effective way.

Another reason for the low level of prevention is that people do not adapt to it. The EuroAspire investigation has shown that even in a high-risk group the adaptation of healthy lifestyle is very limited and disappointing after discharge from rehabilitation. Alternative motivaton concepts are needed. In order to encourage and maintain a preventive lifestyle, scientific, technical and psychological challenges can be identified:

- The scientific challenge is to find solutions for prevention and early diagnosis.
- The technical challenge is to develop solutions that allow ubiquitous access to medical expertise for empowering the citizen to adapt a healthy life style and early diagnose of acute events.
- The psychological challenge is to create pleasant and easy to use solutions that motivate people to adapt their lifestyle and improve their quality of life.

It is the objective of MyHeart to address these three challenges in one integrated project.

2. Scientific Objective: Solutions for Prevention and Early Diagnosis

The MyHeart approach for solving the key challenges is based on the development of intelligent biomedical clothes for preventive care applications tailored to specific user groups. In order to focus on the user motivation and the individual benefit, we define the main objectives along 5 different application areas. These application areas reflect the main risks for developing a CVD and address the user need for early diagnosis to limit the severity of an acute event. The five identified application areas are:

2.1. CardioActive: Application cluster for improved physical activity

Physical inactivity is a major risk factor for developing a cardiac disease and 57% of the European citizens follow a sedentary lifestyle. People must be made aware of this, and stimulated to be more active. For this group we develop solutions for determining the activity levels including the assessment of the fitness condition of the user. The solutions include the assessment of basic vital signs like heart rate, breathing rate and activity classification. Specific training plans and recommendations for training will be personalised on the individual condition and the ambition level of the user. Specific attention is paid on the motivation to stay active by feedback on status, community building and virtual competition.

2.2. CardioBalance: Application cluster for improved nutrition and dieting

More than 20% of all European citizens suffer from obesity defined by a body mass index exceeding 30. For these citizens we develop solutions to actively manage their dieting and nutrition by personalised dieting plans, continuous feedback, guided physical training plans. We work on location dependant services to guide the user for healthier food, e.g. salad bars, special dieting restaurants or point of sales. Special attention is paid to the motivation of the customer via community building and new methods of electronic peer pressure.

2.3. CardioSleep: Application cluster for improved sleep and relaxation phases

More than 25% of all European citizens suffer from sleep disorders, like sleep apnea and insomnia. These patients are at elevated risk to develop a cardio vascular disease. We develop solutions for assessing the individual sleep quality and the diagnosing of sleep disorders at home. We explore novel methods for improving sleep quality and the therapy of sleep disorder based on biofeedback and personalised relaxation exercises. Special attention is paid for diagnosing sleep quality related diseases like depression, which is a frequent complication of post myocardial infarction patients.

2.4. CardioRelax: Application cluster for improved solutions to deal with stress

Stress is a major behavioural risk factor for CVD and more than 40% of all European citizen suffer from stress. We develop solutions not only for diagnosing acute stress events and a stress meter but we also develop specific relaxation methods to deal with stress. Biofeedback tools are used tailored to individual needs and enabled by Web and mobile services. The solution will limit the stress related risk for CVD and will improve the personal performance in the working environment.

2.5. CardioSafe: Application cluster for early diagnosis and prediction of acute events

For early diagnosis we develop solutions to continuously analyse the vital signs of the user in order to determine acute events and predict acute events. We develop diagnosis system for:

- Myocardial infarction: The objective is to detect myocardial infarctions and ischaemic events. In case an ischaemic event is diagnosed an immediate alarm is sent via mobile or fixed networks to an emergency service.
- Stroke Prevention: 15 % of all strokes are due to atrial fibrillation (AF). Our strategy is to diagnose and treat AF to reduce the overall incidence of stroke. For the detection of AF we develop an automated diagnosis tool and derive individual self-therapy recommendations.

- Pump Failure Prevention: The approach is to monitor high-risk congestive heart failure patients and detect early indicators for pump failure. Early diagnosis will allow to direct the user to institutional points of care for further treatment.
- Sudden Cardiac Arrest (SCA) Prevention: The consortium develops methods to detect VT episodes, elongation of the QT interval and other early indicators for sudden cardiac arrest. By this method we can effectively identify people at risk for sudden cardiac arrest. After diagnosis, implant therapy or ablation therapy can be used to prevent SCA in this risk group.
- Hypo-Hyperglycaemic shock: The continuous measurement of ECG, breathing rate and activity are used to develop solutions to detect and potentially also predict hypoglycaemic events. The user will be effectively empowered to prevent an event by self-medication.

3. Technical Objectives: Intelligent Biomedical Clothes for Monitoring, Diagnosing and Treatment

It is the aim of the MyHeart project to develop innovative, personalised, easy-to-use solutions and tools, which help the citizen to adopt permanent healthier lifestyle. A prerequisite for recommendations to change is to get information about the current health status and lifestyle of the user. Therefore we develop solutions that will continuously monitor vital signs and context information, diagnose and analyse the health status and acute events, provide user feedback and seamlessly provide access to clinical and professional expertise if required. For continuous measurements, we develop electronic systems that are embedded into functional clothes with integrated textile and non-textile sensors. Intelligent clothes are able to continuously monitor vital signs, make diagnosis and trend detection and react on it (therapy recommendations). Intelligent clothes have integrated wireless technology to link to user feedback devices and if necessary to professional medical centres.

3.1. Technical Objective 1: Continuous Monitoring

The first basic requirement of preventive lifestyle and early diagnose of acute events is a continuous monitoring of the cardio-vascular system. We will solve this challenge by the integration of novel sensors and monitoring systems into functional clothes. We research and develop a basic set of clothes that allows the continuous monitoring throughout the day.

Three garments serve the full spectrum of prevention as described in the scientific objective:

- Garment for the night (night-dress, pyjama),
- Garment for the day (functional undergarment)
- Garment for sports (functional fitness dress)

Through this focus, we can cover nearly 100% of a user's life with this limited set of garments.

This set of functional clothes comprise innovative fabric sensors for ECG, breathing rate, galvanic skin, response, blood circulation and trans-thoraic impedance.

In addition we develop electronic systems integrated into the functional clothes. This on-body electronics is flexible, bendable and washable and offering the same look-and-feel experience as normal clothing. The on-body electronics adds additional sensors for the detection of movement, the detection of context information (e.g. Global Positioning System location) as well as sensors for blood pressure and oxygen saturation. The system not only allows the acquisition and storage of data, but also the online analysis of the data and provides the needed processing power for diagnosing the health status. Wireless technology is used to connect the system to wired and wireless communication infrastructure and to acquire data from external sensor and intelligent (home) environments.

3.2. Technical sub-objective 2: Continuous Personalised Diagnosis

The intelligent biomedical clothes will provide a modular basis for an on-body diagnosis system that allows for the first time the continuous assessment of the health status and the diagnosis in a wearable on-body system. The personal sensor signals are analysed and high quality diagnosis of the health status is enabled. One of the major challenges of the project is the development of these personalized diagnostic and trend detecting algorithms and the technology to operate these diagnostic algorithms in wearable electronics. By the implementation of clinical protocols and clinical knowledge into the continuous on-body diagnose system we will provide access to clinical excellence on a life-long timescale and in a continuous way.

3.3. Technical sub-objective 3: Continuous Therapy

The intelligent biomedical clothes provide information on the actual health condition. Therapy can be provided in form of specific user instructions and information. Examples are on-line recommendations during sports to control heart rate and breathing rate. The dynamic posture and gesture recognition will allow home training and physical therapy in the home setting under supervision. Biofeedback technologies are developed for stress and relaxation exercises. Personal treatment recommendations and feedback on the success of activities represent a tool to motivate citizen to continue their preventive lifestyle. We explore and research opportunities for a novel self-medication approach for e.g. pill-in-the-pocket.

3.4. Technical sub-objective 4: Feedback to user

We develop and adapt end user terminals that allow the visualization of recommendations and biofeedback in the home and in the mobile setting, anytime and anywhere. We focus on existing platforms and infrastructure like GSM and 3G networks in the mobile setting and on existing home infrastructure like TV, PC and audio-systems. Health status as well as instructions for adapting the lifestyle and notifications of preventive actions will be displayed automatically on mobile terminals as well as on connected home devices. Special emphasis is on ease-of-use aspects, especially for elderly people.

3.5. Technical sub-objective 5: Remote Access and Professional Interaction

Innovative interactive communication systems connect the user to medical professional services and to other users in the home and mobile setting. We explore architecture and concepts for direct and immediate access to institutional care anytime, anywhere. There is need for application specific modules that enable professionals the interaction with MyHeart applications. Moreover, tools for the management of the MyHeart system from external site as well as interfaces of the MyHeart platform with general and third party resources have to be developed.

4. Measurement of Results

The key scientific objective is to develop the MyHeart system to motivate citizen to adopt a healthier lifestyle and to use the system to enable early diagnosis. Hence the success of the project is critically dependent on the acceptance and adoption by the end user. In addition we have to show the medical effectiveness and to demonstrate cost benefits compared to the classical health delivery system.

The MyHeart project starts from the application point of view. We have identified five application clusters Cardio-Active, Cardio-Sleep, Cardio-Relax, Cardio-Balance, and Cardio-Safe. These five application clusters address the risk factors inactivity, sleep-disorders, stress, inadequate nutrition that can be fought by prevention and the detection of acute events such as heart attack.

In order to tailor these applications towards the specific needs of users we introduce the definition of concepts, see Figure 2. Concepts are applications that are tailored to a specific user group or customer segment. Within the first phase of the project, 16 potential concepts are investigated and worked out. For the development of each of the 16 concepts the following 5 'basic questions' have to be addressed and answered:

- What is the application / value proposition?
- Who is the customer / user?
- How to do it technically?
- How to proof feasibility and user acceptance of the concept?
- What is the business?

At the end of the first phase there will be a detailed concept description, a clear business plan and first feedback from users and service providers. The feedback is obtained by showing early mock-up systems that clearly indicate the concept's potential impact and benefits.

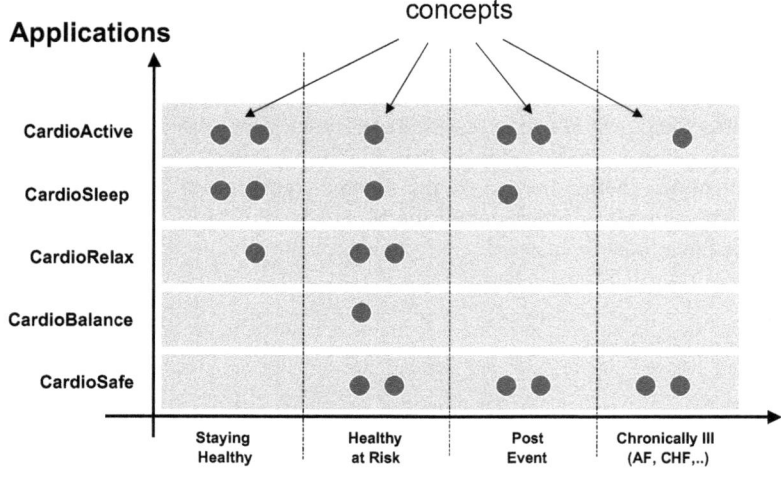

Figure 2. Definition of concepts for tailoring application areas to specific user requirements.

The introduction of concepts allows us to implement the application for a specific customer / user group, see Figure 3, and test the technical feasibility and the user acceptance in this targeted group. In phase 1, the project tests 16 different concepts via a portfolio approach.

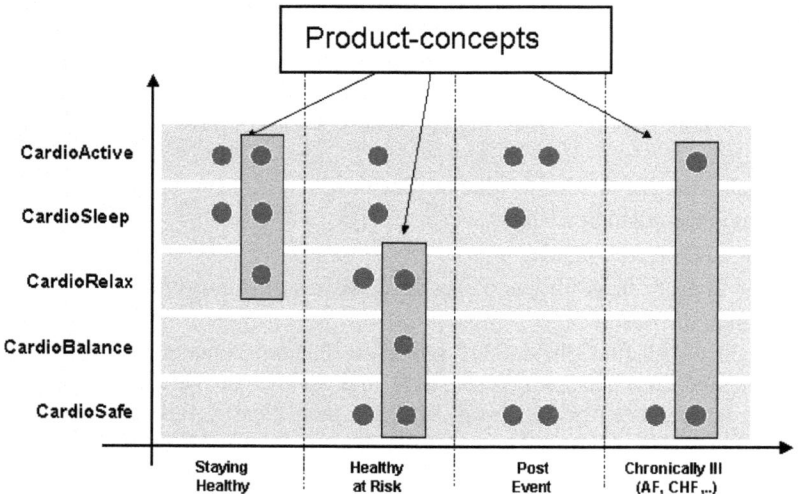

Figure 3. Product-concepts represent combinations of concepts for a specific user group

5. Project Phases

In **Phase 1** (Month 01-18), we implemented basic functional prototypes and tested these concepts in interviews. The definition of concepts also enables us to assess the validity of each concept with relevant stakeholders from the medical domain and from payers like health insurance, employers, pension funds and specific user groups and boards. This intense co-design with users is a key innovation element addressing the main risk of user/stakeholder acceptance. The outcome of this assessment will be used to validate business plans for each individual concept and will be used to select the most promising concepts for further technical and business development in the next phase.

In **Phase II** (Month 18-30), MyHeart will select and combine the most successful concepts and define three to five product concepts. These product-concepts are tailored to specific customer groups and can be composed of several concepts e.g. for post myocardial infarction patients we might combine some concepts out of different application area's like activity, sleep management with early detection of acute events. (Product concepts = combination of different application concepts for one specific user group). These product-concepts are prototype descriptions of future MyHeart products. These product-concepts will be implemented and tested in clinical environments to show the effectiveness and feasibility in long-term test beds. On top of that, the product concepts will undergo a second iterative process of focus group assessment with end-users, professional service providers and medical professionals.

In **Phase III** (Month 31-45) the consortium will validate the product-concept in extensive test-beds and trials for long-term follow-up to show the effectiveness of the product concepts. With long-term test beds we will show that users will use the system over months and years and we will document the success in terms of adaptation of healthier life-style and in the reduction of acute events. The consortium intends to do the testing and trials with control arms to objectively document the advances in quality of care, quality of life and cost benefits. We will benchmark against clear outcome parameter like weight reduction, reduction in average heart rate, reduction in blood pressure, increase in physical activity and in the reduction of hospitalisation days for acute events. The outcome will be documented in improvement of the quality of care delivered to the participants.

In addition we will assess the cost benefits for the stakeholders in the health care delivery system. The final outcome includes documented test beds showing the effectiveness and efficiency and the design of business models for exploitation of the results. We will put special emphasis on novel methods for reimbursement and derive financials benefits for users.

Acknowledgement

MyHeart is a European project funded by the European Commission in the 6th framework (IST-2002-507816).

II. Smart Textiles

Personalised Health Management Systems   63
C.D. Nugent et al. (Eds.)
IOS Press, 2005

Motion Aware Clothing for the Personal Health Assistant

Gerhard TRÖSTER[1], Tünde KIRSTEIN[1], Paul LUKOWICZ[2]

Wearable Computing Lab, ETH Zürich, Switzerland[1]

Computer Systems and Networks, UMIT Innsbruck, Austria[2]

www.wearable.ethz.ch

Abstract This paper sketches the vision and first results of a 'Personal Health Assistant' PHA, opening up new vistas in patient centred healthcare. The PHA is comprised of a wearable sensing and communicating system, seamlessly embedded in daily clothing. Several on-body sensors monitor the biometric and contextual status of the wearer continuously. The embedded computer fuses the vital and physiological data with activity patterns of the wearer and with the social environ-ment; based on these data the on-body computer generates the 'Life Balance Factor' LBF as an individual feedback to the user and to the surroundings afford-ing effective disease prevention, management and rehabilitation, the last also involving telemedicine. The state-of-the-art enabling technologies: smart textile technology and miniaturization of electronics combined with wireless communication, along with recent developments in wearable computing are presented and assessed in the context of multiparameter health monitoring.

Keywords. wearable computing, context recognition, personal health assistant, life balance factor, smart clothing.

1. Personal Health Assistant

Driven by cost and quality issues, the health systems in the developed countries will undergo a fundamental change in this decade, from physician-operated and hospital centred health systems to consumer operated personal prevention, early risk detection and wellness systems.

Andy Grove, Intel's legendary founder, has characterized the current situation of healthcare using the metaphor of mainframe computers, the dominating systems in the sixties [1]: few, expensive powerful machines, localized in a dedicated environment and operated by skilled specialists acting as interface between the user and the computer. Personal computers in the eighties, and mobile phones and PDAs in the nineties have outstripped mainframes in quantity and performance. Could we imagine a similar trend, from mainframe healthcare to a personal health assistant PHA?

Recent developments in micro- and nano-technology, low power computing, and wireless communication as well as in information processing have paved the way to non-invasive and mobile biomedical measurements and health monitoring [2] providing the technological platform for the PHA.

The PHA should be continuously available, seamlessly embedded in our daily clothing, enabling extended perception, providing context-aware functionality as well as proactive support in information processing, perpetually active in a wide range of mobile settings [3].

Figure 1 depicts a potential implementation of a PHA. Several smart miniaturized sensors, distributed in the clothes, transmit the measured physiological and contextual data over a body area network (BAN) to a computing unit (e.g. a PDA), which extracts the relevant parameters, estimates the health status and communicates with the surrounding networks.

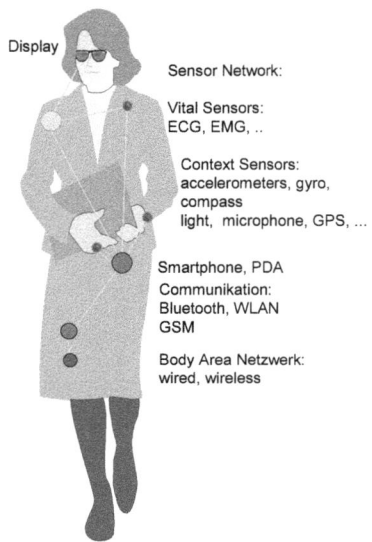

Figure 1. Structure of a 'Personal Health Assistant' PHA.

2. Life Balance Factor

A scenario may help to illustrate the potentials of the PHA. The PHA monitors continuously the wearer's vital signs such as heart rate, heart rate variability, temperature and motion activities. The combination of vital parameters with the wearer's context, their activity and sleep patterns, social interactions and other health indicators paint a picture of their physiological state. To facilitate the interface between the PHA and the individual user the authors propose a 'Life Balance Factor' LBF as a simple health measure and gener-ally understandable indicator, especially designed for medical laypersons. The LBF represents the current physiological state; it indicates health changes and can be used to trigger a consultation with a health specialist if parameters surpass normal range.

3. User's Context

The concept of context awareness constitutes the crucial feature of personal healthcare systems: only by fusing the data on the status of the user with that on their surroundings will a reasonable comprehension of the vital parameters be possible.

Several attributes are considered in context awareness, e.g. the user context, the environ-mental context and the social context. The user context comprises e.g. the user's motion and activity, gestures, biometric data and health status parameters including the affective and emotional state such as stress and depression. The location, both indoor and outdoor, the time, the weather, the illumination and noise characterise the environmental context. The social context includes the people in the surroundings, the contact and communication with them.

As described below, context recognition relies on the sensor data. In [4] recommendations are presented on which sensors or combination of sensors are most appropriate to detect specific context components. Several methods and tools have been proved for data fusion, feature extraction and classification as depicted in Figure 2. The Bayesian decision theory offers a fundamental approach for pattern classification. Nonparametric techniques like the k-nearest neighbour approach enable the design of decision functions based only on sample patterns. The Kalman filter or the recently proposed particle filter approach [5] are helpful tools for tracking and monitoring of states such as hand gestures in video sequences. Hidden Markov Models and the Viterbi algorithm are appropriate to estimate a sequence of decisions. The adaptive and learning properties qualify multilayer neural networks for context recognition by training with repetitive presentations of the target values, e.g. motion patterns.

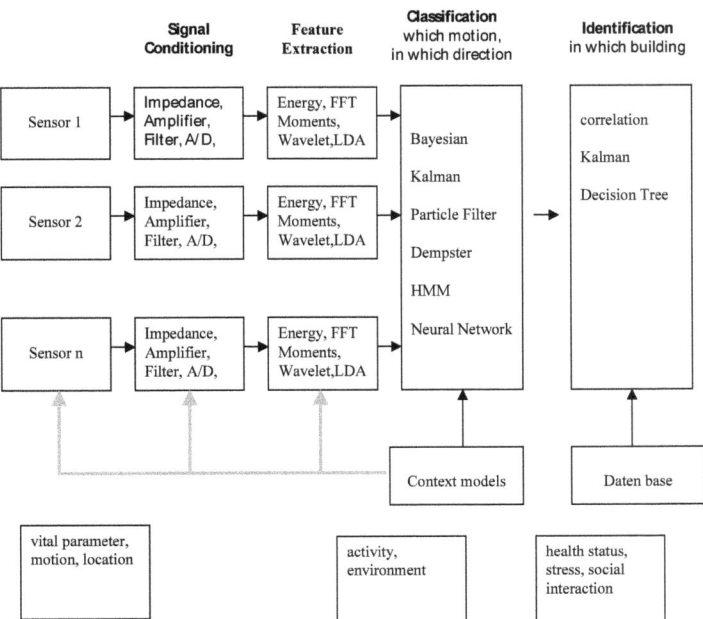

Figure 2. Context recognition data path.

3.1. Activity

Motion, motion pattern, gestures and postures are basic elements characterising human activity. As described above, accelerometer, gyroscope and compass sensors are available in miniaturised and wearable forms, being precise enough to enable the detection of complex motion patterns. As proved in [6], body-mounted inertial sensors can acquire the kinematics of gait with a precision comparable to optical-based, stationary motion capture system. These wearable sensor platforms make the detection of physiologically relevant motion patterns possible. For example [7], an accelerometer system, fastened by an elastic waist belt to the subject's back in the lumbosacral region, enables assessment of the motor recovery system and of the effectiveness of physi-cal therapy of poststroke hemiplegic (PSH) patients. In [8] a significant correlation between cadence and gait velocity of depressed patients, but not in healthy controls could be verified. The fusion of several sensor data streams can detect even complex gestures as used in the American Sign Language (ASL) for deaf people. In [9] it has been shown, that the combination of a vision system, mounted on the head, and with accelerometers on the wrist could be a promising approach for an automatic ASL recognition system.

3.2. Stress and Emotions

The notion 'Affective Computing' as introduced in [10] describes machines which have the skills to recognise the user's affective expressions, and to respond intelli-gently. These affective expressions include stress, emotions and other psychologi-cal symptoms. Wearable systems afford the noninvasive sensing of physiological patterns. In [11] for example, four wearable sensors (EMG, SpO2, skin conductance, respiration sensor) have been applied to detect and to classify eight different emotions such as anger, grief, joy or hate with a classification accuracy between 60 and 70 percent. Acoustical properties of speech which can easily be recorded by a collar microphone, are well suited as indicators of depression and suicidal risk, as described in [12]. To measure and to evaluate face-to-face interaction between people within a community, a wearable 'sociometer' has been built [13], consisting of an IR transceiver and a microphone. A computational framework extracts socially relevant aspects e.g. identifying dynamics and style of a person's interactions from the raw sensor data.

In past years, notable results in on-line context recognition have been achieved: scenarios in defined setups can be detected with sufficient accuracy. However, these systems are not capable of interpreting arbitrary real-world situations. Progress in multi-modal data processing, in cognitive science and in artificial intelligence could pave the way for wearable systems which understand most real-life scenes.

4. Architecture and Components

The diversity of application fields for wearable computers corresponds to today's variety of system architectures and components, from wristwatch computers [14] to robust smart survival clothing for arctic environments [15]. Our daily clothing, optimised over several centuries, has a hierarchical structure. The underwear physically contacting our skin has to fulfill high requirements concerning hygiene and comfort. The outer clothing levels are exposed to the environment. We select them according to our personal preferences and business, mostly divided into garments we wear constantly, and garments like a coat we change several times during the day. The authors have proposed the System-on-Textile (SoT) integration concept for wearable computers, which takes into account the structure and functionality of our clothes [16]. The wearable computer is partitioned into four functional levels: functional textiles, embedded microsystems, attachable peripherals and standard mobile components as depicted in Figure 3.

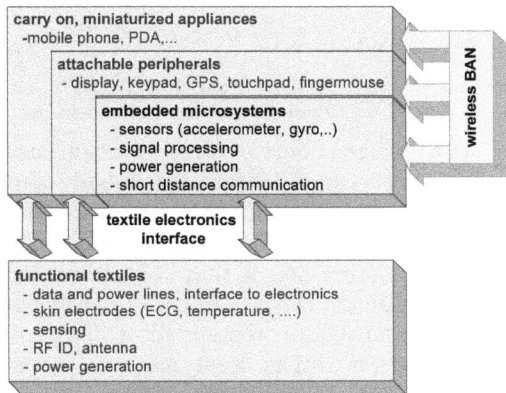

Figure 3. The architectural levels of the PHA.

5. System on Textile

For wearable computing, textiles can provide information and power transmission capabilities, sensory functions and an infrastructure for embedded microsystems.

5.1. Functional Textiles

Originally developed for antistatic applications, conductive textiles can act as an interconnection substrate for electronic systems substituting cables in clothes. Figure 3 shows an example of a woven conductive fabric [17]. Measurements confirm that these conductive textiles are suitable for data transmission [17]: more than 100Mbit/s can be transmitted over a distance of 1 meter, sufficient for a textile body area net-work (BAN). The performance remains unchanged even if the textiles are creased and stretched.

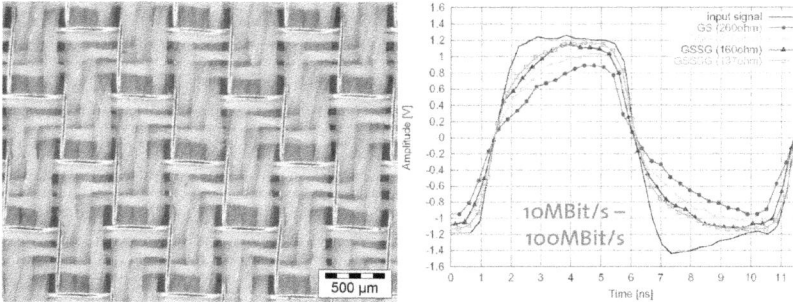

Figure 4. a) Matrix woven fabric with metal fibers (Sefar™) , b) 100 MHz clock signals measured through four different 20 cm long textile transmission lines.

Antennas. Besides wired connection, wireless communication channels are also necessary to enable the data exchange between the on-body components and the user's environment. For the body-area network BAN several communication schemes are available. Magnetic induction with textile coils can effectively bridge distances less than 2 cm, e.g. between trousers and a shirt. Figure 5a shows an application of magnetic induction, the connection between the MP3-player box and the earphones in the shirt. Similar approaches have been proposed for textile transponder systems (RFID tags) [18]. Magnetic induction suffers from the low power efficiency at longer distances. Figure 5b shows a novel textile antenna for Bluetooth applications, which can be sewn into garments. Three textile layers form this circularly polarised antenna [19].

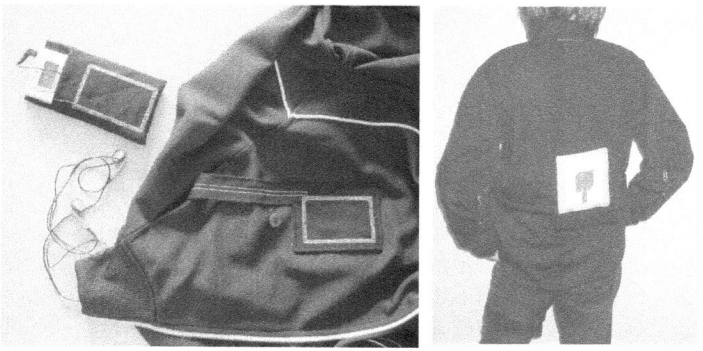

Figure 5. a9 Wireless connection using sewed textile coils, b) textile Bluetooth antenna.

5.2. Embedded Microsystems

As described below, knowledge of the user's context is an essential feature in user-centered healthcare systems. The heterogeneity of possible contexts necessitates the data fusion of various sensor outputs. Vision and speech recognition are established tools of mirroring the human perception, but context detection using vision and speech creates a high computing load. The use of different, simple sensors can reduce the communica-tion and computational effort [4]. To provide sufficient signal quality, most sensors need to be positioned at a particular body location, often in direct contact with the wearer's body or the environment. As a result of the progress made in microsystem technologies over the last decade, many sensors have become small enough to be integrated into our daily clothing. . last decade,

Several technologies, are becoming available for the embedding of microsystems, either directly into fabrics, or into clothing components like buttons. As a design example [20], Figure 6 shows an autonomous sensor button, consisting of a light sensor, a micro-phone, an accelerometer, a microprocessor and a RF transceiver. A solar cell powers the system even for continuous indoor operation.

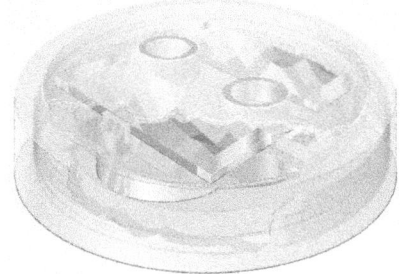

Figure 6. Design of an autonomous 'sensor button' , diameter 15mm, height 5mm.

5.3. Attachable Peripherals

Add-on modules, attached to our clothes and using the textile infrastructure tailor the functionality of the wearable computer to user needs and user situations. d gestures are suitable to allow control of a computer without losing contact with or the environment. Miniaturised microphones fit into collars in a snowboard jacket, as already presented.

5.4. Appliances

The fusion of the mobile phone, PDA (Personal Digital Assistant) and even MP3 player into 'smartphones' offers an interface between the personal communication environment and public services including the Internet. Additionally the 'smartphone' can be connected to components in clothing using e.g. the Bluetooth communication system. Today's 'smartphones' require manual handling and focusing on the interface. Stripped of bulky IO interfaces and large batteries, mobile computing and communication modules are small enough to be easily carried in a purse or be part of carry-on accessories such as a key chain or a belt buckle as depicted in Figure 7 [21].

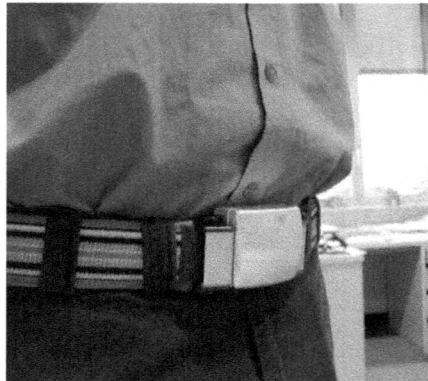

Figure 7. ETH-QBIC – a mobile computer (Xscale CPU, 256 MB SRAM, USB, RS-232, VGA, Bluetooth) integrated in a belt buckle; the belt houses the flexible batteries and interface connectors.

6. Outlook

The wearable 'Personal Health Assistant' PHA is an unobtrusive platform for individualised health service and will be the key enabling technology driving the paradigm shift from established centralized medical care to user-centred overall life-style health management. The proposed 'Life Balance Factor' LBF compiles the current physiological state and translates it into layperson's language. What could be the main road blocks and problems to be solved on that way? Smart clothes pose two critical challenges: On the one hand, the acceptance of the potential users to put the smart clothes on daily requires a high level of wearing comfort and intuitive handling. On the other hand, cooperations between clothing manufacturers, electronic suppliers and retail outlets have to be established to complete the manufacturing, trading and maintenance chain. Furthermore, the PHA as a mobile and communicating device has to be embedded in the local and national IT landscape, involving the net provider, as well as private and public health services. Finally, probably the most critical problem due to the necessary interplay between many partners with partly conflicting interests, is the PHA must also to be integrated into the well-established health organisations, including the family doctor, caregivers, first aid organizations, drug manufacturers, pharmacies, hospitals, and completing, the health insurance agencies. Taking into account all these manifold challenges, the ongoing projects in academia and industry indicate that we will see the first commercially available PHAs in two to three years from now.

References

[1]   Schlender B. Intel's Andy Grove: The Next Battles in Technology. Fortune, 12 May 2003: 80-81.
[2]   Lymberis A. Smart Wearables for Remote Health Monitoring, from Prevention to Rehabilitation: Current R&D, Future Challenges. Proc of the 4th Annual IEEE Conf on Information Technology Applications in Biomedicine. UK, 2002: 272-275.
[3]   Pentland A.Wearable Intelligence, Scientific American, Fall 1998, vol. 9, no 4.
[4]   Lukowic P, Junker H, Stäger M, von Büren T, G. Tröster G. WearNET: A Distributed Multi-Sensor System for Context Aware Wearables. Proc. of the UbiComp2002, Springer, 2002: 361-370.
[5]   Doucet A, de Freitas N, Gordon N. Sequential Monte Carlo Methods in Practice. Springer: 2000.

[6]   Mayagoitiaa RE, Neneb AV, Veltinkc PH. Accelerometer and rate gyroscope measurement of kinematics: an inexpensive alternative to optical motion analysis systems. Journal of Biomechanics 35;2002: 537–542

[7]   Akay M, Tamura T, Higashi Y, Fujimoto T.Unconstrained Monitoring of Body Motion During Walking. IEEE Eng. Medicine and Biology Mag. May /June 2003: 104-109.

[8]   Lemke MR, Koethe NH, Schleidt M. Timing of movements in depressed patients and healthy controls. Journal of Affective Disorders 56; 1999: 209–214.

[9]   Brashear H, Starner T, Lukowicz P, Junker H. Using Multiple Sensors for Mobile Sign Language Recognition. Proc. ISWC 2003: 45-52.

[10]   Piccard RW. Affective Computing. MIT Press 1997.

[11]   Picard RW, Vyzas E, Healey J. Toward Machine Emotional Intelligence: Analysis of Affective Physiological State. IEEE Trans. Pattern Anal. Mach. Intelligence, vol. 32, Oct 2001: 1175-1191.

[12]   France DJ, Shiavi RG, Silverman S, Silverman M, Wilkes DM. Acoustical Properties of Speech as Indicators of Depression and Suicidal Risk. IEEE Trans. Biomed. Enf. vol. 47; July 2000: 829-837.

[13]   Choudhury T, Pentland A. Sensing and Modeling Human Networks using the Sociometer. Proc. ISWC 2003: 216-222.

[14]   Narayanaswami C, Kamijoh N, Raghunath M, Inoue T, Cipolla T, Sanford J, Schlig E. IBM's Linux Watch: The Challenge of Miniaturization. IEEE Computer, Jan 2002: 33-41.

[15]   Rantanen J, Alfthan N, Impiö J, Karinsalo T, Malmivaara M, Matala R, et al. Smart Clothing for the Arctic Environment. Proc. ISWC 2000: 15-23.

[16]   Lukowicz P, Kirstein T, Tröster G. Wearable Systems for Health Care Applications, Methods Inf Med, 3/2004: 232-238.

[17]   Cottet D, Grzyb J, Kirstein T, Tröster G. Electrical Characterization of Textile Transmission Lines. IEEE Trans. Advanced Packaging, vol 26; May 2003: 182-190.

[18]   Kallmayer C, Pisarek R, Cichos S, Gimpe S. New Assembly Technologies for Textile Transponder Systems. Proc. ECTC May 2003.

[19] Klemm M, Locher I, Tröster G. A Novel Circularly Polarized Textile Antenna for Wearable Applications. European Microwave Conference, Amsterdam, October 2004.

[20]   Bharatula NB, Ossevoort S, Stäger M, Tröster G. Towards Wearable Autonomous Microsystems. Pervasive 2004, Springer; 2004: 225–237.

[21]   Amft O, Lauffer M, Ossevoort S, Macaluso F, Lukowicz P, Tröster G. Design of the QBIC wearable computing platform . Proceedings 15th IEEE Int. Conf. on Application-specific Systems, Architectures and Processors, ASAP 2004.

Personalised Health Management Systems
C.D. Nugent et al. (Eds.)
IOS Press, 2005

Integrated Microelectronics for Smart Textiles

Christl LAUTERBACH, Rupert GLASER, Domnic SAVIO, Markus SCHNELL,
Werner WEBER
Infineon Technologies AG, Corporate Research, Munich, Germany

Abstract. The combination of textile fabrics with microelectronics will lead to completely new applications, thus achieving elements of ambient intelligence. The integration of sensor or actuator networks, using fabrics with conductive fibres as a textile motherboard enable the fabrication of large active areas. In this paper we describe an integration technology for the fabrication of a "smart textile" based on a wired peer-to-peer network of microcontrollers with integrated sensors or actuators. A self-organizing and fault-tolerant architecture is accomplished which detects the physical shape of the network. Routing paths are formed for data transmission, automatically circumventing defective or missing areas. The network architecture allows the smart textiles to be produced by reel-to-reel processes, cut into arbitrary shapes subsequently and implemented in systems at low installation costs. The possible applications are manifold, ranging from alarm systems to intelligent guidance systems, passenger recognition in car seats, air conditioning control in interior lining and smart wallpaper with software-defined light switches.

Introduction

Many promising technologies are emerging in the area of intelligent textile materials like electrically conductive yarns or pressure sensitive fabrics. State of the art feature sizes of integrated circuits allow for powerful and yet small and cost-effective microelectronic devices. Many interesting applications in the field of technical textiles arise by merging micro-systems and textile fabric structures [1]: pressure sensors in floor coverings for alarm systems or motion detection (person tracking), indicator lights in floor or wall coverings for guidance systems in public buildings, distributed sensor networks for detection of defects in textile concrete constructions, and many more.

Approaching the given task of electronics integrated into large areas, the following questions arise: How can we exploit the functionality of all the integrated microprocessors, sensors and light emitting diodes? What happens, if the smart fabric is cut to fit as e.g. a functional floor covering in an arbitrarily shaped room? Will a single destroyed or defective module or wire lead to a complete failure of the function of the smart textile system? To address these problems we decided to use a self-organizing and fault-tolerant architecture for the integrated sensor network. Research on self-organizing systems is presently pursued extensively, worldwide [2]. Several years ago, we developed ADNOS (algorithmic device network organization system) for building a self-organizing and fault-tolerant wired peer-to-peer network for large sensor and actuator areas [3]. Our first demonstrator of this technology is the "Thinking Carpet" described below.

In previous work Paradiso et al. [4] describe a "Magic Carpet", where an array of piezoelectric wires and Doppler radar motion sensors are used to track the motions of a performer in musical installations. Orr and Abowd [5] use a single pressure sensitive tile within the "Smart Floor" for identification of persons by their characteristic foot pressure profile during walking. In contrast, by using ADNOS we achieve a homogenous touch-sensitive floor, which is capable of self-installation and automatically circumvents defective areas of the sensor network. Moreover, through the localization of the sensor signals, speed and direction of the movement can be analyzed and trigger software-defined events in the PC application.

1. Smart Textile Concept

Figure 1 shows a schematic of the smart textile. The modules are connected to each of their four neighbors. One of the modules is connected to the PC and used as the portal. As depicted, several defects may occur within such a wired peer-to-peer sensor network during fabrication or use: open lines, destroyed or missing modules and electrical short circuits. High yield and robust functionality require fault-tolerance for all those defects. In addition, the demand for simple and low-cost installation requires that the smart textile can be cut into irregular shapes to fit into any given room.

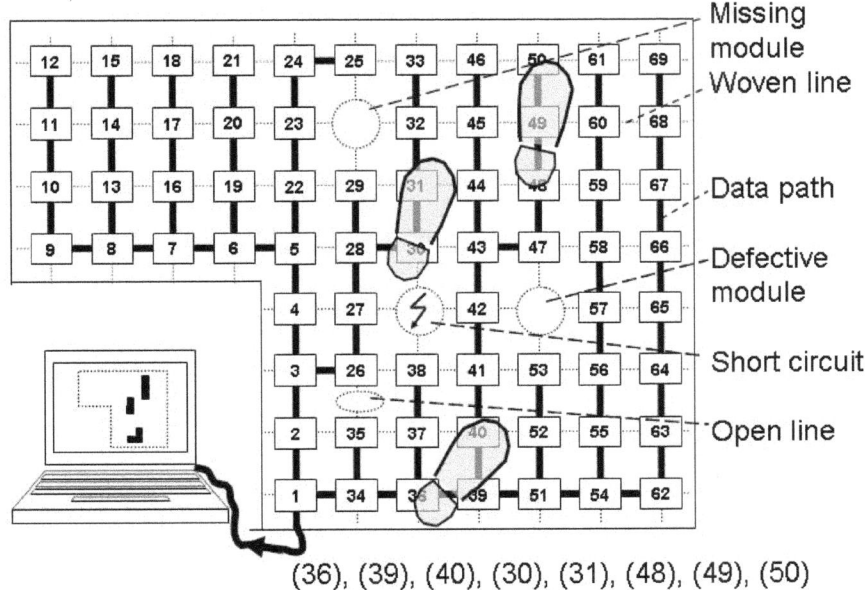

Figure 1. Schematic of the wired network within the "smart textile", showing the automatically numbered modules and routed data paths; the indicated possible defects can be handled by ADNOS; sensor data are sent to the PC via the portal.

2. Textile Integration of Microelectronics

The smart textile (Figure 2) is based on a polyester fabric with interwoven silver-coated copper wires. Three of these wires with a diameter of 70 μm are spun to one cord. For redundancy and low line resistance four cords are used for each line. The pitch of the woven pattern is 20 cm in weft and warp directions, respectively. The width of the textile is six pitches or 120 cm. Each ADNOS module is connected to its four neighbors by two supply and two data lines. Two additional lines per module are used as sensor lines for the touch sensor. To achieve a larger sensitive area of the touch sensor, we embroider a meander-shaped wire. The modules are connected at the crossover points of the conductive lines in a single step using anisotropic-conductive adhesive (Figure 2 right). The achieved contact resistance is 7 mΩ/contact. At the crossover areas the conductive weft and warp fibers are removed to eliminate the electrical shorts of the interwoven conductive wires. The modules are encapsulated before mounting to reduce mechanical stress.

conductive fibers

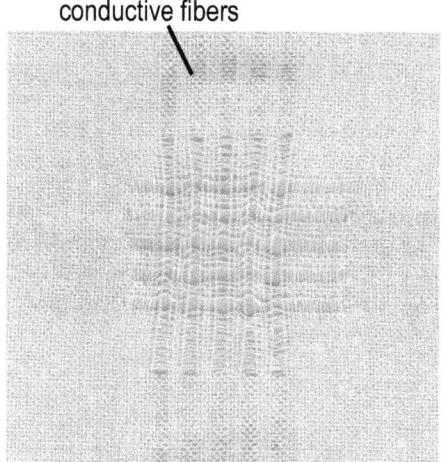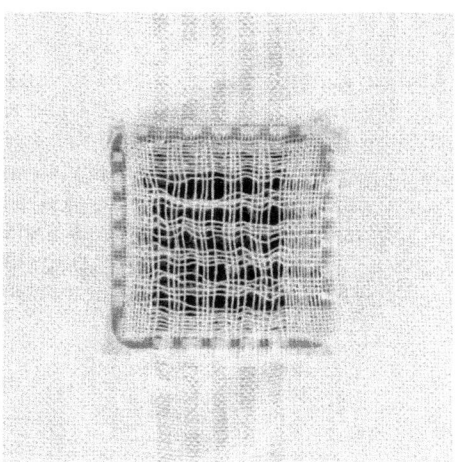

Figure 2. Crossover area of the conductive wires (left), the wires are removed before bonding the module, bonded module with contact areas (right) ADNOS module.

3. ADNOS Peer-to-Peer Network

Each ADNOS module has four UARTs as ports to the connected neighbors and the input of the capacitive touch sensor (Figure 3). The power supply of the textile uses a voltage of 12 V in order to decrease the distribution losses. It is reduced to 3.3V at the module by a switched power supply. For the demonstrator we use a commercially available 16 Bit microcontroller. 18kB Flash and 4kB RAM are sufficient for our system. The modules are active during data transfer, only. Their power consumption is approximately 10 mA/module at 12 V in active and 6 mA/module in standby mode.

Within the network each module exchanges control messages with its four neighbors and controls and drives a specific region. No prior knowledge about their position within the grid is used. The control data are fed into the network by a functional block referred to as *portal*, which is connected to an arbitrary module at the edge of the array.

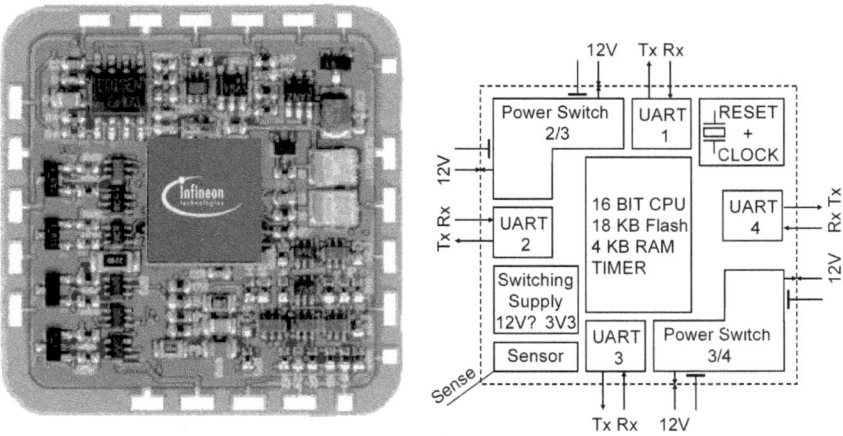

Figure 3. Photograph of the ADNOS module with a size of 3.5 cm x 3.5 cm (left) and the corresponding block diagram (right).

A set-up phase is started in each module as soon as it is connected to the power-supply. During this phase, called "power routing", short circuits within the network are detected and affected branches switched off. The power switches at each module are able to switch up to 1.25 A. Their resistance is below 150 mΩ. In larger networks we prefer to use several power inputs uniformly distributed along the edges of the network.

Next, the self-organization of the network according to the ADNOS rules is started by the PC. Every module computes the positions of its neighbors. The portal starts this process by feeding the absolute position to the first module. In the next phase the minimum distance to the portal is computed by each module sending its own estimated distance to its neighbors. Based on the previously computed data, routes are generated, that will later carry the data stream (Figure 1). The portal then starts an automatic numbering based on the established routes and the calculated throughput through each module. This enables the modules to determine a unique address number. The generated address number format yields sufficient routing information for each module. Except for the address numbers of its direct neighbors, no additional routing tables are needed inside the network. If new defects occur, the self-organizing routine can be repeated and new routing paths emerge in the network.

The ADNOS algorithms establish a peer-to-peer communication scheme, which is used to transfer data between the modules and between the network and the "smart textile" monitor application on the portal PC, respectively. The four ports of each module have different priorities. On simultaneous reception on two ports (messages received within 8 μs), the port with the highest priority will accept data first. To avoid an unbalanced response of the network, the priority of ports is regularly rotated. Below the ADNOS layer a protocol layer is responsible for communication between neighboring modules. To accommodate data collision, reception and transmission are performed in full duplex mode. The board layer takes care of hardware control and physical connection between neighboring modules.

The sensor data from the network are transmitted to the "smart textile" monitor application. We use an RS232 interface at a data rate of 115200 bps. The customized features are defined within the monitor application, e.g. processing and evaluation of sensed data or control of light-emitting diodes.

Figure 4 shows the PC user interface of the "smart textile" monitor. All recognized modules, the functional connections between the modules and the established data paths are depicted in the left area of the screen. Sensor events are represented by highlighted dots at the connected module. The pattern shown in Figure 4 was produced by a person walking from the lower left to the upper right of the smart textile. All information gained within the network during the self-organization like coordinates, address, throughput, distance to the portal, etc. can be depicted on demand on the screen.

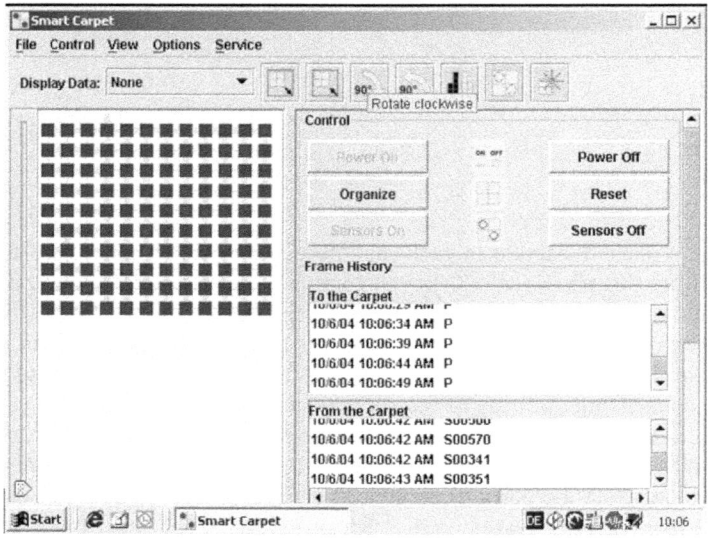

Figure 4. Screenshot of the ADNOS user interface on the PC featuring a "smart textile" network with 120 integrated modules (left side). The white dots indicate the sensor signals produced by a person walking from the lower left to the upper right edge of the textile.

4. Results

To illustrate the functionality of the ADNOS system we fabricated a demo board with twelve modules. Figure 5(a) shows a photo of the demo board with pluggable modules and three screen shots of the ADNOS user interface on the PC (b-d). The modules are depicted as dark squares. The broad lines are established data paths, thin light lines are connections not used as data paths. Figure 5(b) shows the screen shot of the network with all modules plugged in. In Figure 5(c) one module in the middle of the network has been removed as shown in Figure 5(a) to simulate a defective module. ADNOS has recognized the failure (marked dark) and shows, that all modules connected to the same data paths are no longer contributing to the functionality of the network (the color changed to light). After initializing the reorganization a new data path is found surrounding the missing module (Figure 5(d)). All remaining modules are fully functional again.

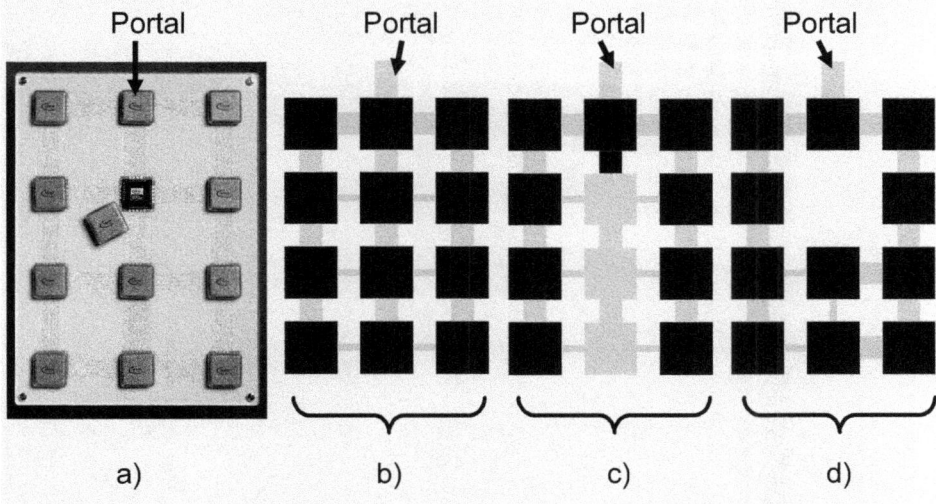

Figure 5. ADNOS demo board with twelve pluggable modules (a) and three screen shots (b-d) of the ADNOS user interface on the PC, (b) original network, (c) one module removed and failure recognized by ADNOS, (d) after reorganization.

The maximum size of the network for a single power supply can be calculated from the measured results derived from our smart textile demonstrator. The cumulated resistances in the network are 0.4 Ω/m for the interwoven copper wires and 7 mΩ/contact for the interconnect to the interwoven copper wires. The on-resistance of the FET switches is 150 mΩ. The standby current of one module is 6 mA at 12 V. For the supply voltage we use a switched power supply with 85 % efficiency at 12 V. The network is fully functional down to 8 V. At the usual width of a carpet of 4 m the voltage drop is 1.1 V at a pitch of 20 cm (20 modules) and 0.25 V at a pitch of 50 cm (8 modules). To calculate the delay time of the smart textile network we measured the delay between hops of the network as a function of the number of hops from a stimulated sensor of a module to the portal. We find an average time of 1.6 ms per hop, independent of the distance from the PC portal. An additional delay of approximately 1.6 ms will be added if data collisions occur at one module. However, the probability for simultaneous data reception (time <8µs) is very low.

5. "Thinking Carpet" Prototype

The integration technique of the smart textile in a carpet was developed in cooperation with the carpet manufacturer Vorwerk-Teppich and presented at the Orgatech 2004 in Cologne, Germany.

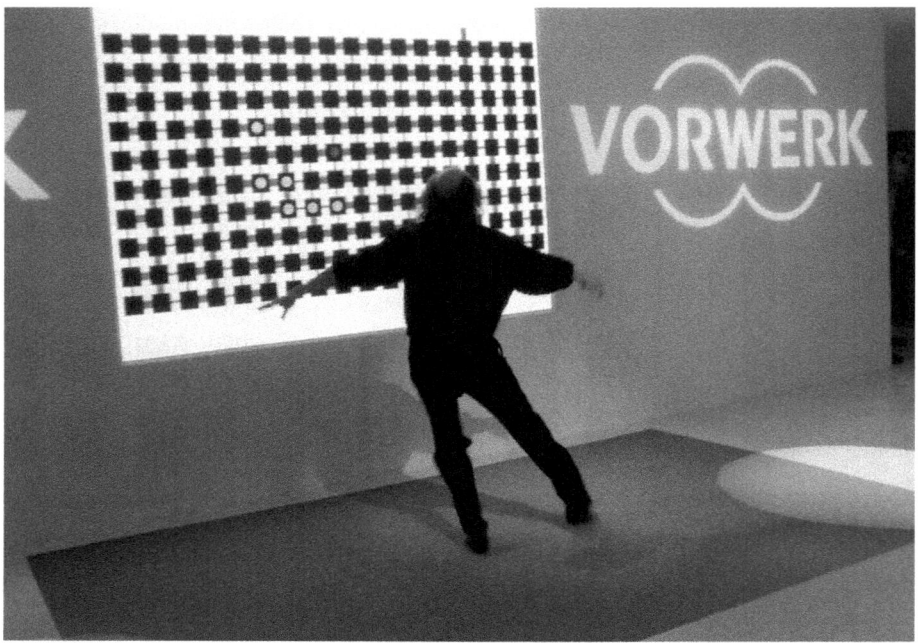

Figure 6. "Thinking carpet" installation at the Orgatech 2004 (darker rectangle at the floor), featuring 180 ADNOS modules with capacitive sensor areas. The display on the back plane shows the recognized modules. The light dots indicate sensor signals produced by the dancer.

Using the technology described above, four "thinking carpet" prototypes were fabricated with 60 integrated modules and a size of 120 cm x 220 cm, each. The smart textile was cold-laminated between two layers of textile to reduce the mechanical stress and equalize the height of the modules (2 mm). The top layer is a tufted carpet combined with a 1000 g fleece as backside. The power consumption of each carpet is 8.0 W. For the Orgatech prototype three carpets were connected to each other, therefore forming one single network. Figure 6 shows a photograph of the "thinking carpet" taken at the Orgatech. The touch sensitive floor is the darker rectangle in the photograph. The large display at the back plane shows that all 180 integrated modules are recognized. A closer look at Figure 6 reveals open lines between several modules. However, due to the ADNOS self-organization, new data paths were established surrounding the defects. All modules and sensors are fully functional. The light dots shown at the display are sensor signals produced by the dancer.

The integrated capacitive touch sensor is fully functional through an insulating layer up to 30 mm thickness. Therefore all usual flooring materials like wood, stone, concrete, ceramic or glass can be used on top of the smart textile.

6. Application Scenarios

The customized features are defined within the PC application, e.g. how the sensor data are processed and evaluated, or how light-emitting diodes are controlled. Interesting examples for new applications are smart textiles working as alarm systems in the flooring of private or public buildings, in tents or truck tarps. Textile reinforced concrete with an integrated ADNOS network could automatically detect cracks after an earthquake.

An interesting application is the smart floor in apartments for elderly or handicapped people. Different functions can be triggered using data mining on the sensed data: The light will be switched on automatically, when a person enters the room or steps out of bed. If a person doesn't leave the bed for an unusually long period, a nurse will be called. Doors will open and close automatically, when the person moves towards it. If a person falls down on the floor and doesn't move afterwards, an emergency call will be activated. Such functionality would give elderly or handicapped persons a chance to live a self-determined life without running an intolerably higher risk in case of an emergency.

Security applications in public or private buildings are of increasing interest. Statistical evaluation of the sensed data derived from the smart floor will distinguish "normal" behavior of airport users from unusual behavior of possible terrorists. Security areas will be defined within the software application. Having for example information about speed and direction of movements, footsteps starting from the window side of a building will trigger a burglar alarm.

In the future, the ADNOS functionality will be integrated into a single silicon chip with an estimated chip size of approximately 7 mm² using a 180 nm CMOS process. A density of four modules per m² seems sufficient for smart floor applications, when using larger sensor areas. The range of suitable and available sensors and actuators is wide-spread: sensors are available for various parameters such as pressure, temperature, humidity, smoke, gas, and sound. Integrated light-emitting diodes will give the possibility to build large-area displays, thus achieving intelligent guidance systems or flexible displays.

References

[1] Marculescu, D., Marculescu, R., Zamora, N. H., Stanley-Marbell, P., Khosla, P. K., Park, S., Jayaraman, S., Jung, S., Lauterbach, C., Weber, W., Kirstein, T., Cottet, D., Grzyb, J., Tröster, G., Jones, M., Martin, T., Nahkad, Z.: Electronic Textiles: A Platform for Pervasive Computing, Proceedings of the IEEE, Vol. 91, No. 12, 2003, pp. 1995–2018.

[2] Di Marzo Serugendo, G., Karageorgos, A., Rana, O. F., Zambonelli, F.: Engineering Self-Organising Systems, ISBN 3-540-21201-9, Springer-Verlag Berlin Heidelberg, 2004.

[3] Sturm, T. F., Jung, S., Stromberg, G., Stöhr, A.: A Novel Fault-Tolerant Architecture for Self-organizing Display and Sensor Arrays, 2002 SID Symposium Digest of Technical Papers, Volume XXXIII, Number II, 2002, pp. 1316–1319.

[4] Paradiso, J., Abler, C., Hsiao, K., Reynolds, M.: The Magic Carpet: Physical Sensing for Immersive Environments, Proceedings of the CHI '97, Conference on Human Factors in Computing Systems, Extended Abstracts, ACM Press, NY, 1997, pp. 277–278.

[5] Orr, R. J., Abowd, G. D., The Smart Floor: A Mechanism for Natural User Identification and Tracking, Proceedings of the CHI '00, Conference on Human Factors in Computing Systems, The Hague, Netherlands, 2000.

Personalised Health Management Systems
C.D. Nugent et al. (Eds.)
IOS Press, 2005

Wearable Sensors? What is there to sense?

Sarah BRADY[a]*, Lucy E DUNNE[b]*, Aogan LYNCH[a]*, Barry SMYTH[b],
Dermot DIAMOND[a]

[a]*Adaptive Information Cluster, National Centre for Sensor Research,*
Dublin City University, Dublin 9, Ireland
[b]*Adaptive Information Cluster, Department of Computer Science,*
University College Dublin, Belfield, Dublin 4, Ireland
**These authors contributed equally to this work.*

Abstract   This paper provides an overview of research conducted in the development of ambulatory devices for wearable sensing applications. Two configurations of wearable sensing are shown, the first a wearable chemosensor in a wrist-watch configuration, and the second a textile with an integrated foam sensor. The foam sensor is composed of polypyrrole-coated polyurethane foam, which exhibits a piezo-resistive response when exposed to electrical current. The potential of wearable sensing is discussed using these examples to illustrate the relevant concerns.

Keywords: wearable sensors, ambulatory devices, conducting polymers, miniaturisation.

Introduction

We live in a world of information, and emerging technologies compel us to look for new ways to collect, process, and distribute information. Today we are faced with a significant information overload problem as users struggle to locate the right information in the right way at the right time. In response to this issue, a number of researchers have suggested that adaptive information technologies may hold the key to the next generation of ubiquitous information systems; i.e., systems that automatically adapt to changes in their environment and usage in order to deliver a more intelligent, proactive and personalised information service. In this paper we provide an overview of the issues involved in producing practical wearable chemosensors and physical transducers.

1. What are the Issues with Wearable Sensors?

Computerisation impacts every aspect of modern life and society, but as we know, computers are most adept at processing digitised data. This data must be collected, stored if required, and transferred to a computer from which useful content can be extracted, processed and interpreted. Increasingly, sensors are the source of data used by networked systems and in the case of wearable devices, it is often advantageous for sensors to be fully integrated into textiles, or common wearable objects, rather than attached in semi-conventional form to the body, garment, or textile surface. In the context of wearable systems, monitoring is required in numerous situations and can be categorised as either;

- "Inward Looking", e.g., to measure state and activity of the user, including movement, activity, and vital signs such as ECG, cardiac frequency, respiration, blood oxygen saturation, or as
- "Outward Looking", i.e., to measure parameters in the surrounding environment, for example in emergency/disaster situations, or in extreme environments as may arise during military actions and space experiments, and in certain sports, such as mountain climbing.

In all cases, however, it is desirable that the availability of information regarding the physical condition of the wearer, or his/her environment, should not compromise the comfort of the wearer. Traditional sensing technologies are rarely designed for continuous, on-body use: those that require skin contact are generally designed to be used in a hospital or doctor's office, and those that do not are generally designed for use in stationary devices. Consequently, the achievement of certain design goals for existing sensors (such as durability) is almost always detrimental to the user's comfort when applied to the wearable environment. For example, in many cases durability often equals stiffness, which results in a solid-state device that can cause discomfort by localising pressure.

2. Wearable Sensors

If sensors are to successfully integrate into the user's peri-personal space, then their structural and aesthetic form should fit the individual's preferences and essentially "disappear". The form adopted by the sensors is application dependent. Non-invasive sensors are the most promising innovations for the monitoring of daily activities, offering painless and comfortable applications. However, a major issue arises with ready access to well characterised samples. It is unfortunate from the wearable sensor perspective that the best sample for diagnostics is blood, as this implies that the chemo/bio-sensor must be implanted, or in direct contact with blood that is drawn to a wearable external device through a catheter or shunt sampling system. In practice, all existing chemo/bio-sensors suffer a limited effective lifetime (at best, a number of weeks) and during this time they must be regularly recalibrated to produce accurate results. Furthermore, direct contact with blood over extended periods of time invariably results in infection.

Other potential sample sources for wearable chemo/bio-sensors include faeces, urine, saliva, sweat, intracellular fluids, tears, and breath [1]. While some diagnostic tests have been developed for saliva, and many exist for urine, access to the sample remains a problem. There is potential to design a wearable device that samples breath, particularly within the virtually enclosed environment provided by Emergency-Disaster (E-D) clothing. The most easily accessible sample fluid is sweat, but there is limited knowledge of its diagnostic capabilities. One device we have examined is a wearable 'watch-sensor' incorporating chemical sensors that can measure diagnostic markers in sweat. The device is worn on the wrist in the normal manner over a region previously stimulated using pilocarpine iontophoresis to generate sweat. Sweat trapped between the base of the 'watch' and the skin is drawn into the device through a narrow flexible tube and within a few minutes comes in contact with electrochemical sensors embedded in the device which can monitor the electrolyte composition of the sweat (see Figures 1 and 2). We have particularly focused on sodium and chloride concentrations which are diagnostic for Cystic Fibrosis (CF) [2], and demonstrated that the wearable sensors can reduce the test time from half a day, to less than one hour (including the pilocarpine stimulation phase). Furthermore, the test can be performed at point of need, rather than at a specialist center that has the complex bench-top instruments typically used for this test. In a limited clinical trial, the device successfully discriminated between CF positive and normal samples (Figure 3).

The wrist-watch configuration is advantageous in that it is robust and mobile and can be readily accepted as a wearable device. At the wrist, parameters such as skin temperature, skin electrical conductance and potential, blood oxygen saturation, sweat analysis and heart rate can be measured [3], for example during sports activities [4]. The miniaturisation and integration of functions such as sensing, signal processing and communications makes it possible to produce a device such as an innocuous 'smart' wrist watch, capable of monitoring general health and well-being, therefore making these diagnostics more readily acceptable to the user. However, incorporation of chemical sensors and biosensors for long-term use is currently beyond the state-of-the-art and commercially available devices are focused on monitoring physical parameters that are general indicators of well-being such as blood pressure [5]. Nevertheless, devices incorporating biomedical sensors and actuators in principle have enormous potential [6] and are in some cases generating a paradigm shift from "cure" to "prevention" and from "hospital-based healthcare" to "point-of-need diagnosis" [7].

The success of the Cystic Fibrosis study highlights many of the issues impeding the introduction of longer-term wearable diagnostics such as;

- Access to a sample fluid that contains diagnostic markers but does not lead to infection of the wearer during extended use, e.g. sweat test for CF diagnosis or urine for pregnancy testing.
- Calibration of the chemo/bio-sensing device – in the above case, the device initially contains a calibration solution, which is displaced by the sample. Furthermore, the above example is a 'single-shot test', which is successful because it does not involve continuous use over extended periods of time. For long-term wearable chemo/bio-sensors, calibration will be a difficult issue as it implies regular access to standards.
- Stability and reliability of the sensor – chemo/bio-sensors invariably suffer from drift, as they depend on a chemo/bio-active surface whose characteristics change with time, and in many cases, malfunction or "biofouling" will happen within a relatively short period of time (typically days). This is avoided in our example by choosing a 'single-shot' application and discarding the sensor after use, a common practice in many clinical tests.

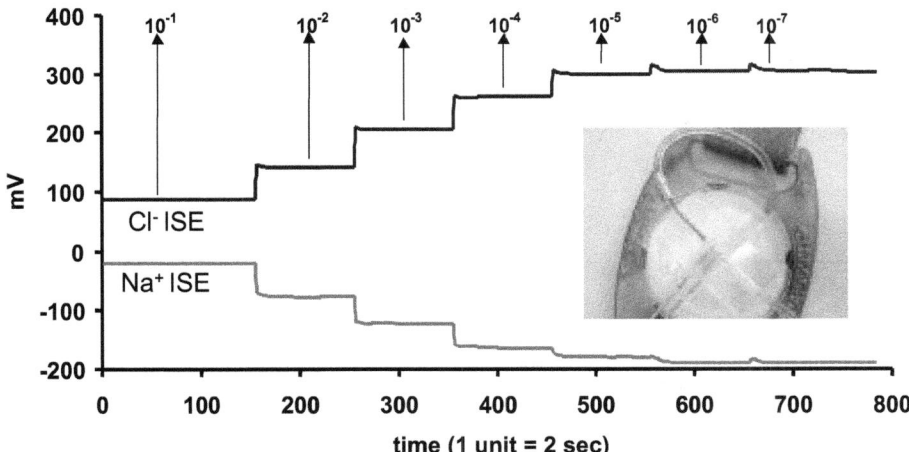

Figure 1: Wrist-watch configuration for point-of-need diagnosis of cystic fibrosis [2]; Repeat calibration runs of sequential 10-fold dilutions of 0.1 M NaCl measured with a sodium PVC-membrane ion-selective electrode [8] and a bare Ag/AgCl wire electrode. Theoretical (Nernstian) response should be ca. 60mV per dilution step. Inset picture shows sweat (dyed blue for easy visualisation) filling the sampling tube and contacting the integrated electrodes.

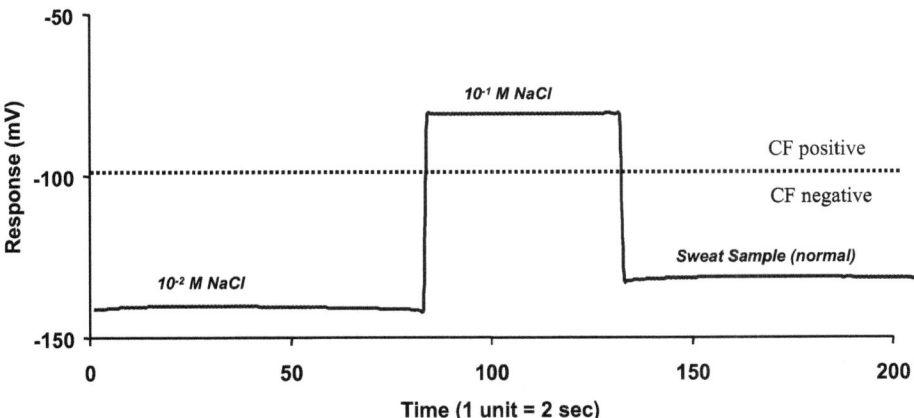

Figure 2: Performance of wearable sweat analyzer shown in Figure 1. Data shows responses to two calibration solutions (10^{-2}M and 0.1 M NaCl) followed by a real sweat sample. The decision line for positive vs. negative is shown. The device correctly classified the sample as negative.

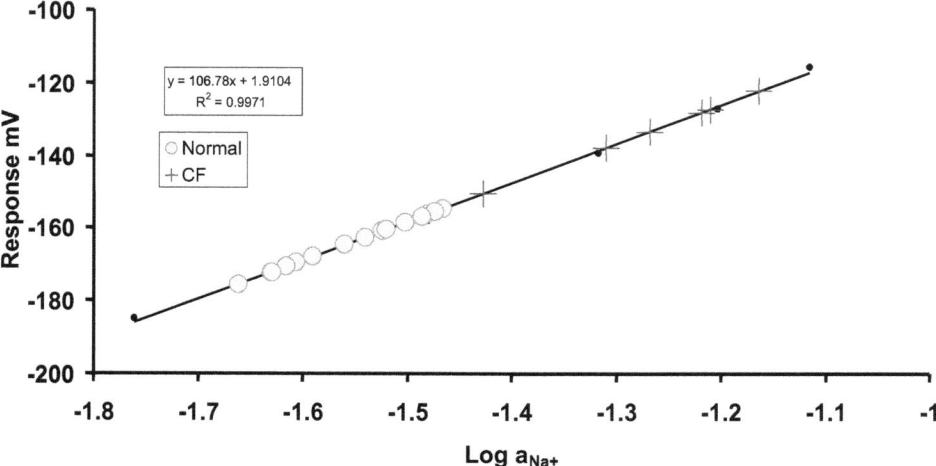

Figure 3: Results of Smart Watch study showing ability to discriminate between CF positive and normal samples using the Na-ISE signal only

3. Smart Textiles

One of the possible short-comings of these types of wearable sensors is the limited physiological parameters that may be measured due to the reduced contact area between the body area, for example, the wrist or finger, and the device. One solution to these limitations could be the integration of sensors into a wearable platform that has a large area of contact with the body. This notion of an unobtrusive sensory system suggests that smart or intelligent textiles may provide the solution – the key issue is how to make a textile that has an inherent sensing capability. Many textile-based sensors are actually fabricated by coating a textile with a sensing material [9] or by forming sensing materials into fibres which are woven or knitted into a textile structure [10]. The specifications of the ideal textile-based sensor are extremely challenging, as they integrate those of the textile such as flexibility, washability, stretch, and hand (texture of textile) with the electronic properties required for the sensor, which include durability, power consumption, and ease of connection into a circuit. Metallic components, designed to function in rigid environments, often do not satisfy these needs. For instance, a metallic element in a high-flex environment (such as a garment) will soon break. However, the recently discovered conducting electroactive polymers (CEP), offer a potential solution to this problem [11]. CEPs such as polypyrrole (PPy), polyaniline and polythiophene constitute a class of polymeric materials that are inherently able to conduct charge through their polymeric structure. They can be reversibly switched from the doped conducting state to the undoped insulating state upon chemical or electrochemical treatment. In particular, polypyrrole has attracted much interest because it is easily prepared as films, powders and composites, has a relatively high conductivity and is relatively stable in the conducting state. However, when the black precipitate of PPy has been formed it is insoluble to all known solvents and is non-processable. To overcome this PPy can be simultaneously polymerised and deposited onto the substrate [11]. The result is that the substrate is covered with a thin layer of Ppy, rendering the whole object conducting without compromising the mechanical properties of the substrate [12, 13].

In previous work [14], a novel polymer synthesis methodology was developed to create a textile-like structure capable of sensing changes in planar or perpendicular pressure, by coating an open-cell polyurethane (PU) foam with a CEP (polypyrrole). The method involved soaking the substrate, the PU foam, in an aqueous monomer and dopant solution. An aqueous oxidant solution was then introduced into the reaction vessel to initiate polymerisation. This lead to the precipitation of doped PPy, which was subsequently deposited onto the PU substrate. Characterisation of the PPy-coated PU foam was carried out using a number of methods as described in [14]. It was found that by increasing the weight placed upon the PPy-PU foam, or by shortening the overall length of the foam, a decrease in the electrical resistance measured across the foam was observed. Once the foam response was characterised, it was integrated into a garment to explore its performance in a wearable context. The prototypes, including a torso garment (Figure 4), consisted of a number of foam sensors distributed across each garment. The sensor positions were chosen to test the foam reaction to a number of stimuli, including breathing, shoulder movement, and neck movement.

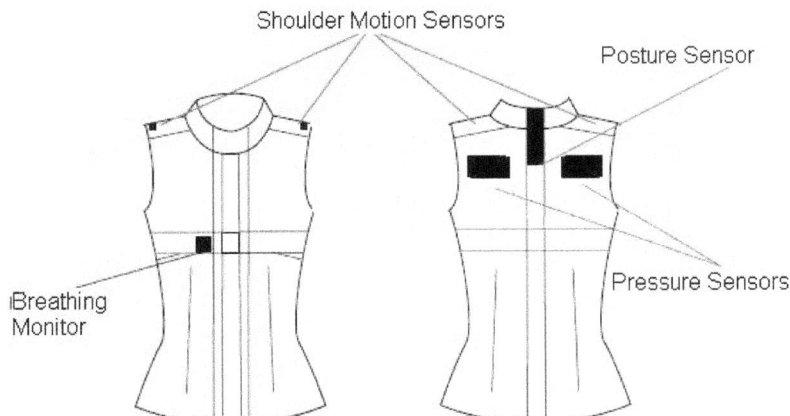

Figure 4 - Prototype pressure sensitive torso garment: Structure and Sensor Layout

Integrating the foam sensors into the torso garment caused little alteration to the visual or tactile properties of the garment. Although comfort was not a measured variable, there appeared to be no change in the tactile comfort of the garment when the sensors were added. In demonstration, both the test subject and other viewers had difficulty locating the sensors within the garment without direction. Results indicated that pressure changes caused by movement could be predictably monitored using this garment [15].

4. Looking Inwards vs Looking Outwards

In addition to monitoring the wearer, it is also important that information about the wearer's environment can exist to alert the wearer to potential dangers and risks. For example during fires, devices that can detect carbon monoxide have a huge potential to reduce fatalities sustained by the fire-fighting profession [16, 17]. Although the materials we have developed so far have focused primarily on monitoring of the wearer, many polymeric materials are known to generate chemically selective signals when exposed to various external target species [18, 19]. For example, it has been found that PPy is up to 10 times more selective towards ammonia than to other common volatiles, see Figure 5. Ammonia may be used as a refrigerant however, it is a toxic irritant, which lead to its replacement by freons. However with the implications of freons in global warming, a move back to ammonia refrigerant may occur. Ammonia is also explosive when combined with air, having a flash point of 11°C. This potentially enables PPy coated textiles to be used for monitoring of the external chemical environment, which can alert the wearer to potential dangers and risks. There are other volatile gases, e.g. explosive gases such as benzene, chloroform, tetrachloroethylene and dinitrotoluene which can be detected with surface acoustic wave devices (SAW) [20, 21]. When miniaturised SAW may be incorporated into ambulatory devices, for on-site environmental monitoring.

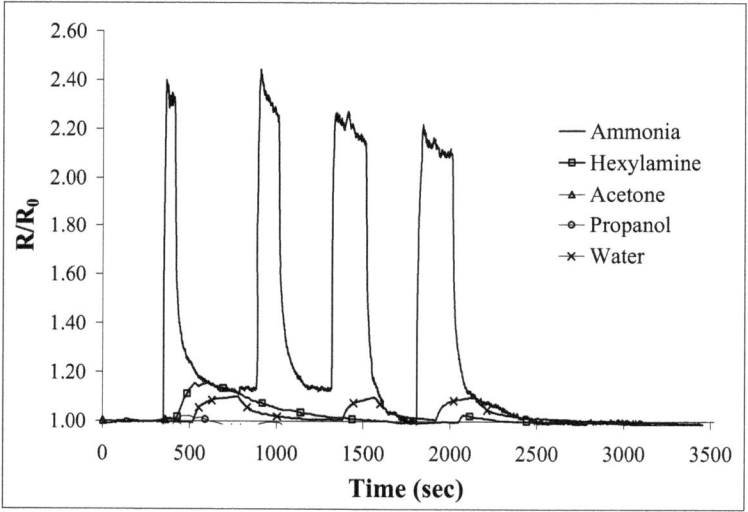

Figure 5 - Relative response of foam sensor to nitrogen samples saturated with the following volatile organic vapours; ammonia, hexylamine, acetone, propanol and water. The large spikes are due to ammonia.

For intelligent textiles, communication may be required within one element of the garment, from the wearer to the garment to pass instructions, or from the garment to the wearer to display information. Currently communications are realised by wires, wireless networks, optical fibres [22], or conductive yarns [23]. Communication with the greater environment can be achieved by the use of wireless communications such as Bluetooth, radio-frequency (RFID) or Zigbee devices [24]. The advantage of integrating antennas into clothing is that a large surface area can be used without burdening the wearer [25]. The development of wearable electronic devices requires a multidisciplinary team approach, and strong collaborations between engineers and scientists from numerous fields, such as mobile and wireless telecommunications, nanotechnology, textiles and apparel, engineering and all general sciences.

5. Conclusion

A radical change in the way global healthcare is organised is clearly needed, in order to tackle the increasing under-delivery of services in the face of escalating costs. At the same time, people are becoming more health conscious and more proactive in their own health management. Given the appropriate tools, people are now prepared to take more responsibility for their own therapy, particularly in conditions that are chronic in nature. Hence demand for pHealth sensors is set to rise, both in terms of general indicators of well-being (e.g. longer term pressure/movement sensors), and short term (single shot in many cases) sensors for specific disease markers. However, issues like calibration and long-term stability remain significant barriers to the integration of chemo/bio-sensors into wearable textiles. Conducting electroactive polymers are attractive for sensing in a garment-integrated context because of their ability to retain the tactile and mechanical properties of a textile-based structure, in contrast to conventionally engineered devices that are attached to a garment.

Outside of medical applications, knowledge of the state of the body is essential in many wearable, mobile, and ubiquitous computing applications. It is common in these applications for a system to make decisions based on its perception of the needs and wants of the user. A range of subtle, comfortable sensors that demand no attention or adaptation from the user can allow such applications to function invisibly, reducing the cognitive load on the user.

Acknowledgements

This material is based on works supported by Science Foundation Ireland under Grant No. 03/IN.3/I361 and IRCSET under Grant No. RS/2002/765-1. We gratefully acknowledge the cooperation of Dr. Gerry Canny, Our Lady's Hospital for Sick Children, Crumlin, Dublin, in the organisation of the Cystic Fibrosis Study.

References

[1]   Mitsubayashi, K., *Wearable chemical sensors and biochemical gas sensors (bio-sniffers) by a soft-mems apporoach.* Annales De Chimie-Science Des Materiaux, 2004. **29**(6): p. 103-114.
[2]   Lynch, A., Diamond, D., and Leader, M., *Point-of-need diagnosis of cystic fibrosis using a potentiometric ion-selective electrode array.* The Analyst, 2000. **125**(12): p. 2264-2267.
[3]   Dittmar, A., Vernet-Maury, E., and Rada, H., *Biometry of the emotional reactivity and vigilance during driving of vehicle and process and sport activity using non-invasive sensors.* Biom Hum Anthropol, 1997. **15**(15): p. 43-53.
[4]   Scheffler M., Hirt E., and Caduff A., *Wrist-wearable medical devices : technologies and applications.* Medical Device Technology, 2003. **14**(7): p. 26-31.
[5]   Asada, H.H., Shaltis, P., Reisner, A., Rhee, A., and R.C., H., *Mobile monitoring with wearable photoplethysmographic biosensors.* IEEE Engineering in Medicine and Biology Magazine, 2003. **22**(3): p. 28-40.
[6]   Dittmar, A., Delhomme, G., and Roussel, P., *Biomedical Micro-sensor and Micro-systems.* REE, 1997. **8**: p. 13-22.
[7]   Lymberis, A. and Olsson, S., *Intelligent biomedical clothing for personal health and disease management: State of the art and future vision.* Telemedicine Journal and E-Health, 2003. **9**(4): p. 379-386.
[8]   Diamond, D., Svehla, G., Seward, E., and McKervey, M., *A sodium ion-selective electrode based on methyl p-t-butyl calix[4]aryl acetate as the ionophore.* Analytica Chimica Acta, 1988. **204**: p. 223-231.

[9]   De Rossi, D., Carpi, F., Mazzoldi, A., Paradiso, R., Scilingo, E.P., and Tognetti, A., *Electroactive Fabrics and Wearable Biomonitoring Devices.* AUTEX Research Journal, 2003. **3**(4).

[10] Hertleer, C., Grabowska, M., Van Langenhove, L., Catrysse, M., Hermans, B., Puers, R., Kalmar, A., Van Egmond, H., and Mattys, D. *Towards a Smart Shirt.* in *Proceedings of Wearable Electronic and Smart Textiles.* 2004. Leeds, UK.

[11] Malinauskas, A., *Chemical deposition of conducting polymers.* Polymer, 2001. **42**(9): p. 3957-3972.

[12] De Rossi, D., Della Santa, A., and Mazzoldi, A., *Dressware: wearable hardware.* Materials Science & Engineering C-Biomimetic and Supramolecular Systems, 1999. **7**(1): p. 31-35.

[13] Munro, B., Steele, J., Campbell, T., and Wallace, G., *Wearable textile biofeedback systems: are they too intelligent for the wearer?* Studies in Health Technology and Informatics., 2004. **108**: p. 271-277.

[14] Brady, S., Diamond, D., and Lau, K.T., *Inherently conducting polymer modified polyurethane smart foam for pressure sensing.* Sensors and Actuators A: Physical, in press.

[15] Dunne, L.E., Brady, S., Diamond, D., and Smyth, B., *Initial Development and Testing of a Novel Foam-Based Pressure Sensor for Wearable Sensing.* Journal of Neuroengineering and Rehabilitation, In Press.

[16] Pescovitz, D., *Smart Dust Sniffers.* Lab Notes, 2002. **2**(6).

[17] El-Sherif, M.A., Yuan, J.M., and MacDiarmid, A., *Fiber optic sensors and smart fabrics.* Journal of Intelligent Material Systems and Structures, 2000. **11**(5): p. 407-414.

[18] Nylander, C., Armgarth, M., and Lundstrom, I., *An Ammonia Detector Based on a Conducting Polymer.* Analytical Chemical Symposium Series, 1983. **17**: p. 203-207.

[19] Dall'Antonia, L.H., Vidotti, M.E., Cordoba de Torresi, S.I., and Torresi, R.M., *A New Sensor for Ammonia Determination Based on Polypyrrole Films Doped with Dodecylbenzenesulfonate (DBSA) Ions.* Electroanalysis, 2002. **14**(22): p. 1577-1586.

[20] Houser, E.J., Mlsna, T.E., Nguyen, V.K., Chung, R., Mowery, R.L., and McGill, R.A., *Rational materials design of sorbent coatings for explosives: applications with chemical sensors.* Talanta, 2001. **54**(3): p. 469-485.

[21] Dickert, F.L., Bruckdorfer, T., Feigl, H., Haunschild, A., Kuschow, V., Obermeier, E., Bulst, W.E., Knauer, U., and Mages, G., *Supramolecular Detection of Solvent Vapors with Qmb and SAW Devices.* Sensors and Actuators B-Chemical, 1993. **13**(1-3): p. 297-301.

[22] VivoMetrics, *LifeShirt.* 2005, Available: www.vivo-metrics.com/site/index.html.

[23] Softswitch. 2005, Available: www.softswitch.co.uk/.

[24] Michahelles, F., Matter, P., Schmidt, A., and Schiele, B., *Applying wearable sensors to avalanche rescue.* Computers & Graphics-Uk, 2003. **27**(6): p. 839-847.

[25] Massey, P.J. *Fabric antennas for mobile telephony integrated within clothing.* in *London Communications Symposium.* 1999. London: UCL.

Personalised Health Management Systems
C.D. Nugent et al. (Eds.)
IOS Press, 2005

Micro and Nano Technology Enabling Ambient Intelligence for P-Health

John BARTON , Sean Cian Ó MATHÚNA, Stephen O'REILLY, Tom HEALY,
Brendan O'FLYNN, Stephen BELLIS and Kieran DELANEY
Tyndall National Institute, Lee Maltings, Prospect Row, Cork, Ireland

Abstract. This chapter will discuss the ongoing development and integration of micro and nano technologies within the Tyndall National Institute that will enable the future vision of ambient intelligence with specific application to the area of personalised health (P-Health). Ambient Intelligent Systems open entirely new possibilities for future applications and resultant markets. Ultimately, these systems will create intelligent environments that cater continuously for the requirements of the individual in everyday life and apply it in a totally coherent manner. They will learn and evolve to anticipate user-requirements. We will discuss ongoing research in the areas of sensors, sensor interfacing, interconnection and packaging, hardware platforms, infrastructure and power delivery for ambient systems with applications in the p-health domain.

Keywords. Micro-nano technologies, ambient intelligence, wireless sensor networks.

Introduction

According to the European Information Society Technologies (IST) Advisory Group, "The concept of Ambient Intelligence (AmI) provides a wide-ranging vision on how the Information Society will develop. The emphasis is on greater user-friendliness, more efficient services support, user-empowerment, and support for human interactions. The Ambient Intelligence environment is capable of recognizing and responding to the presence of different individuals. And, most importantly, Ambient Intelligence works in a seamless, unobtrusive and often invisible way. [1]" Areas like medical monitoring and telemedicine, automobiles, sports, and entertainment are currently beginning to benefit from innovative applications that are building blocks for these AmI systems [2, 3]. From a technological perspective, key requirements for AmI are (1) very unobtrusive hardware, (2) a seamless mobile and fixed communications infrastructure, (3) dynamic, massively distributed networks of collaborative devices, and (4) intuitive, dependable human-computer interfaces that engender trust. Much of the focus of current AmI research is in software development and even concept design.

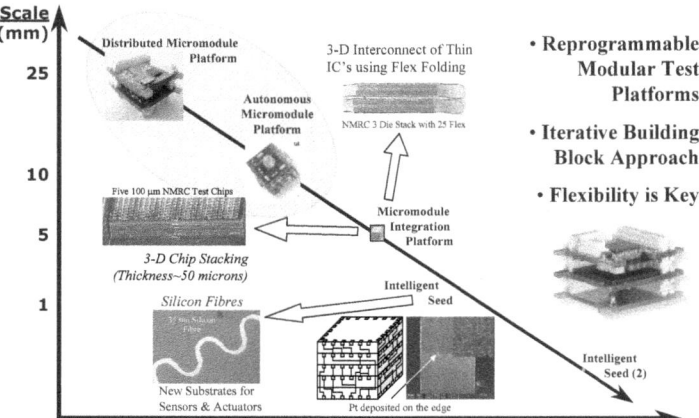

Figure 1. Tyndall National Institute 'I-Seed' Roadmap.

However, significant challenges are present in hardware systems research also. These challenges require significant progress in materials and process development, miniaturisation, new transducer devices, and new integration techniques for scaling systems performance (both in terms of computational capacity and physical size).

The drive to miniaturization and unobtrusiveness will require both the silicon form and function to adapt through increased hybridization with novel integration techniques, and with emerging platforms such as nano-technology. In fact, the importance of this is such that hybridization of micro-nano-systems is seen as one of the major breakpoints leading to implementation of AmI on a global scale.

One of the core research drivers at Tyndall National Institute lies in the development of 3-dimensional and planar microsensor modules that will form the basis of future wireless sensor networks in monitoring systems for sustainable environmental development and diagnostic and therapeutic systems for eHealth, both of which will significantly impact the health of every citizen. Functional elements incorporated in these microsensor modules include sensors, data acquisition and processing, communications and power [4]. This 'Intelligent Seed' programme is about creating appropriate functional architectural templates for enabling AmI, and providing appropriate levels of miniaturisation that solve future production and usability issues. The primary hardware research target that connects these goals is a requirement to develop very highly miniaturised wireless micro-sensor networks of the order of 1mm³ (see Figure 1). This program is guided by a roadmap that incorporates the development of 25mm, 10mm, 5mm, and 1mm cubic modules, each undergoing development and evaluation through selected experimental AmI scenarios. The research is directed towards creating globally scalable, high granularity technology platforms that can be deployed easily and effectively into many types of user environments or embedded into the everyday objects that are used in these environments [5].

The larger 25mm and 10mm cubic formats provide the scope for the rapid-prototype assembly of autonomous transducer systems, serving a critically important purpose in merging hardware, software, and user-design research. Each of these module forms can be viewed as miniaturised, reconfigurable laboratories, and thus as focal points for use in investigating issues such as sensor architecture (e.g. for effectively implementing extrovert gadgets), systems deployment, ad-hoc networks, the integration of intelligence, power management and generation, etc. In terms of purely hardware development these are key factors needing definition, at least as part of a dynamic, iterative process in order to create appropriate targets for functional miniaturisation [6].

The highly miniaturised form factors, 5mm and 1mm Intelligent Seeds, utilize the numerous high-density integration techniques that are the subject of current state-of-the-art research worldwide. In particular, these include multichip modules (MCM), 3-D integration, system-on-chip (SoC), and system-in-a-package (SiP) technology development [7]. Material systems and processes are also being adapted to encompass the changing requirements for very highly integrated autonomous systems. These include the development of very thin flexible multilayer substrates (of the order of 2-3 µm per layer) [8], the integration of thin silicon ICs (each at 50 µm or less), and the development of novel substrates [9] - in particular silicon fibre computing [10] - and new approaches to solve handling and assembly issues for Intelligent Seed modules. The following sections describe research with medical applications and scenarios using these modules as core technology platforms.

1. Wearable Health Monitoring Systems

A key issue in the effective roll-out of eHealth solutions and infrastructure is the development and evaluation of real-life scenarios whereby the deployment of wireless sensor networks can be assessed in terms of delivering benefit to the individual while providing economic value to practitioners in the hospital, the doctor's surgery, the home and the wider community. The following paragraphs present some scenarios that are focussed on gaining an understanding of the issues associated with deployment of wireless sensor networks in an eHealth space.

1.1. Inertial Measurement for Personal Security and Elder-Care Support

Inertial measurement components, which sense either acceleration or angular rate, are being embedded into common user interface devices more frequently as their cost continues to drop. These devices hold a number of advantages over other sensing technologies as they directly measure important parameters for human interaction and they can easily be embedded into mobile platforms.

Case studies have been made into the use of miniaturised inertial measurement units for personal security and in supporting care of the elderly in the home [11]. By connecting the output from the inertial measurement units to a mobile phone, alarm text messages can be relayed in response to a shock (i.e. a fall) or prolonged inactivity (i.e. lack of consciousness). Furthermore, by integrating a Global Positioning System (GPS) system and relaying the text data to a central mapping agency, the exact location and status (in relation to health or security) can support carers and/or emergency services in locating people.

These inertial sensors and others including temperature, bend sensors, respiration, and ECG have been interfaced to Tyndall wireless sensor modules to create a prototype Body Area Network(BAN) which can be relay data wirelessly to a base station e.g. PC,

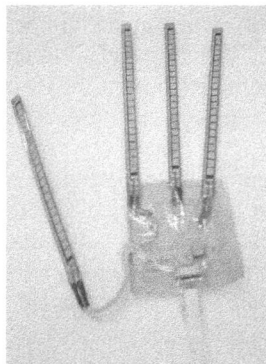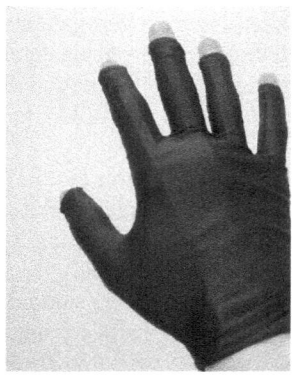

Figure 2. Wearable Sensor Glove before and after integration.

laptop or PDA. Figure 2 shows the sensors fabricated on a flexible substrate located inside a glove. This system can interface with a PC via sign language. These sensors consist of 4 bend sensors and an accelerometer. Next generation of this contains a full 6 Degrees Of Freedom (DOF) Inertial Measurement Unit (IMU) developed as a separate add-on layer for the wireless system [12].

1.2. Sensor Interconnection and Integration

Everyday clothing consists of textile fibres woven and knitted to produce a fabric with the primary purpose being both structural and aesthetic. Fibres can have added functionality by the integration of information technology into the material that forms them. The integration of this IC technology into fibre format is an important development for a wide range of emerging scientific applications from wearable vital sign health monitoring systems to Ambient Intelligence Microsystems. A new concept is proposed [13], which has the potential to change the way advanced circuits and systems are designed and fabricated in the future. The aim is to make large flexible integrated systems for wearable applications by building functional fibres with single crystal silicon transistors at their core. This concept has the potential to provide a planar technology that can be used to manufacture extremely powerful circuits and systems in long narrow fibres, which will create the fundamentals for the realisation of integrating information technology into everyday objects and in particular into high-tech-textile products.

   These fibres have specific applications in anti bacterial functions. A novel concept being developed at Tyndall National Institute in this area is the development of a smart bandage technology. The smart bandage concept offers an exciting alternative to the wearable electronics phenomenon. By combining electric current with other traditional wound healing factors such as antibiotics, an accelerated and efficient wound healing process is anticipated. The concept utilises the electronically functional fibre technology to deliver an electric field across an infected area such as a chronic leg ulcer. One of the key initial considerations involved with this technology is the electrical interconnection of such flexible structures. There are several issues to be addressed within this area including the evaluation of reliability issues associated with connections to the fibres and to the outside world. These connections need to be flexible and robust because the textiles that they are to be included in, are expected to move due to breathing or flexure of joints etc. whilst the circuit is in position and electrically active. With electronically functional fibres it is anticipated that, given that it is washable, heat resistant, and flexible, it would be possible to significantly improve the state of the art in wearable and ambient electronics. The MERMOTH project [14] is currently investigating these interconnection and reliability issues.

1.3. Other applications

RealProf - There are currently some 600,000 prosthesis users and 2.4 million therapeutic footwear users in the EU. Of the worldwide diabetes population of 150 million, 15% will at some point have foot ulceration which can lead to amputation of the foot. The average cost of a 2-year programme of care for each ulcer is 29000 Euro. Currently, there is no means of scientifically monitoring the performance of therapeutic footwear and lower limb prostheses in the real world. This prevents the early detection of problems under the sole of the foot or on the stump that lead to ulceration, and potentially amputation. Also, clinicians prescribing the footwear or prosthesis, and designers of these devices, currently have no means of monitoring the performance of the device once fitted, which is a prerequisite for treatment improvements.

Real-Prof – 'Intelligent Real World monitoring of Prosthesis and Footwear'is an EU [IST-2001-38429] project [15,16], started in January 2003 and lead by the University of Salford, with the aim of developing technologies for monitoring the health of lower limb amputees and patients with orthotic footwear. The core idea behind the project is to identify tissue deterioration in an amputee's stump or in a patient's foot before it progresses too far. The goal is to deliver pre-commercial prototype systems which can monitor patients in real-time, in their everyday life, and transmit data to clinics via secure wireless communication. In this way clinical intervention can occur as soon as problems develop rather than being delayed until the patient's next routine visit to the clinic. Sensors will be integrated into the shoe or prosthesis socket to measure skin pressures, gait motions and other physiological parameters.

MULTIPLEYE - The MULTIPLEYE – (MULTIfunctional PersonaL EYEglass interface) project [17] seeks to develop, characterise and demonstrate a novel display interface that is fully wearable and portable for the delivery of information to users operating in multi-functional contexts. The main applications will be: vision enhancement and navigation in driving, specialised computer assisted operations, office applications, entertainment, infotainment, vision enhancement for visually impaired people, etc. The system will be composed of a primary display source, a compact light-guiding system for the projection of images, a variable-transmittance optical window to allow for different background intensities, a miniaturised inertial system for the tracking of head position and orientation, a radio-frequency Rx/Tx module for the exchange of information between the interface and the base station (including master navigator, image generator), CMOS camera, speakers, microphone, rechargeable battery and driver electronics.

2. Infrastructure

2.1. The E-Ward

The main objective of this work is to assess the feasibility of an ad-hoc wireless network system for use within a hospital. The design is based on a recently developed technology known as eGadgets [18]. An eGadget is an everyday tangible object that: is enhanced with sensing, acting, processing and communication abilities; possesses an ability to cooperate and communicate with other eGadgets and can be connected up in a user-defined wireless ad hoc network known as a GadgetWorld. eGadgets are realised by adding to the object a processor, memory, sensors, actuators and wireless communication module.

This study was undertaken within the EU FET eGadgets project, funded under the Future and Emerging Technologies Disappearing Computer programme. The central aim of the E-Ward section of the project was to implement a medical application that fully exploited the functionality of eGadget technology. The scenario demanded that every bed in a ward be transformed into an eGadget. These so-called eBeds would monitor and record a patient's details including a patient's current condition, a recent record of patient's vitals (e.g. heart rate, body temperature, etc) and a record of patient's medical details and history. (see Figure 3). Appropriate members of the medical staff on the eWard would have a PDA. This PDA would function as an eChart. These eCharts could discover and connect to any eBed in the vicinity. Once discovered, the eChart could view and manipulate information specific to a given patient. While only two different types of eGadgets were developed, namely the eBed and the eChart, multiple numbers of each of these eGadgets exist within the scenario. The only difference between instances of a specific eGadget is their eGadgetID and IP address.

3. Power Delivery for Wearable and In-Vivo Microsensor Modules

A critical issue in the large scale deployment of wireless, ad-hoc, sensor networks is the manner in which each of the nodes can be effectively powered over the lifetime of the application. There is, as with all autonomous systems, a constant trade off between power requirements and the size, weight and type of energy supply. The larger the power requirements and the longer the required operational lifetime, the bigger the power solution required. Striking a balance between lifetime power consumption and the size of the energy solution is nearly always a calculated compromise. We focus on research in the area of inductive coupling.

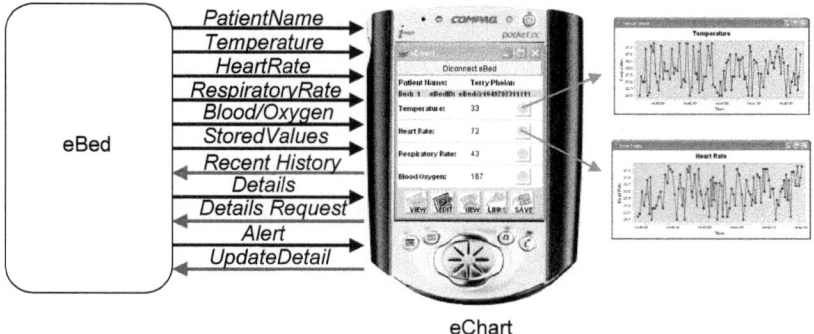

Figure 3. Interaction between an eBed and eChart.

3.1. Inductive Coupling of Power for Biomedical Implants

There are many processes in the human body that, if not functioning properly, could cause long-term discomfort for the individual. Many of these processes/functions could benefit greatly from the use of embedded electronics, thus improving the overall quality of life of the individual. Typical applications are in the area of chronic debilitation through incontinence, diabetes or neural dysfunction.

The objective of the EU project TUBA (Transceiver and Inertial Unit for Biomedical Applications) [19] is to develop key microsystems components for biomedical implants. The system consists of a dual channel inductively-powered, implantable, drop-foot stimulator for stroke victims, see Figure 4. Functional electrical stimulation (FES) is based on the application of current pulses to the peroneal nerve that activates muscle groups that control foot movement during the swing phase of walking. The implant is designed to purely passive (i.e. it contains no active components apart from a rectifier diode) and the external transmitter provides both energy and control through inductive coupling. Planar coils have been developed to replace the actual wire wound version for improved repeatability and reliability. Different coil variations have been implemented in printed circuit board (PCB) and thick film on ceramic technology for the implant. Initial circular spiral inductors have been abandoned due to their poor performance. D-shaped planar coils have resulted in an optimized footprint, an increased inductance range and increased stimulation power. The objective of the MEDPOWER project, funded by Enterprise Ireland under its Technology Development programme, is to develop a platform for the fabrication of highly miniaturised, implantable, rechargeable power modules that will be able to power and control a range of biomedical devices. The proposed module combines the advantages of continuous inductively rechargeable battery power for long-term implants in addition to an inductive, bi-directional communication capability for remote control (state of "health" of the battery) and programming of the circuit, readout of the sensors and alert of the patient before battery runs out of charge.

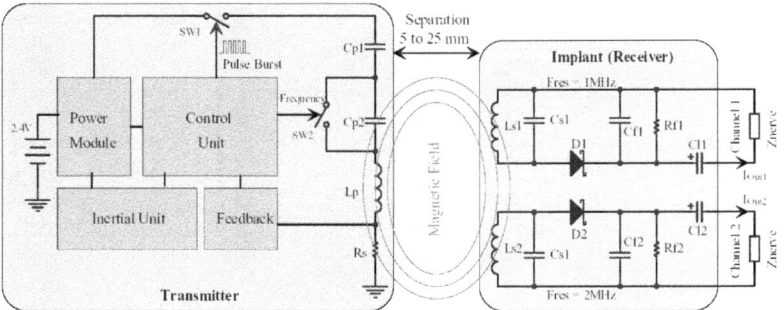

Figure 4. Circuit diagram of the neuromuscular stimulator.

4. Conclusions and Future and Emerging Technologies

This chapter has presented the ongoing development and integration of micro and nano technologies within the Tyndall National Institute that will enable the future vision of ambient intelligence with specific application to the area of personalised health (pHealth). Ongoing research in the areas of sensor development, interconnection and packaging and infrastructure, based around a core group of 3-dimensional and planar microsensor modules has been discussed. Further projects ongoing at Tyndall which may have huge benefits for pHealth include; retinal implants [20], point-of-care DNA analysis systems [21], catheter radiation monitoring [22], and electrochemotherapy for localised cancer treatment [23].

5. References

[1] IST Advisory Group (ISTAG) Scenarios for Ambient Intelligence in 2010: http://www.cordis.lu/ist/istag-reports.htm.
[2] C. O'Mathuna, et al, "MEMS packaging for the Intelligent Environment", Invited presentation at the IMAPS Advanced Technology Workshop, San Jose, Nov 9-12, 2001.
[3] J Paradiso, et al, "Design and Implementation of Expressive Footwear," IBM Systems Journal, Volume 39, Nos. 3 & 4, October 2000, pp. 511-529.
[4] B O'Flynn et al, "The Development of a Novel Miniaturized Modular Platform for Wireless Sensor Networks", 4th Intern'l Conf. on Information Processing in Sensor Networks (IPSN'05), UCLA, Los Angeles, California, USA, April 24-27, 2005 – **ACCEPTED.**
[5] K. Delaney et al, "Creating Systems for Ambient Intelligence" – chapter in "Silicon: Evolution and Future of a Technology" pubs Springer-Verlag Berlin 2004, eds, Siffert and Krimmel, pp 489-514.
[6] J Barton et al, "Development and Characterisation of Ultra Thin Autonomous Modules for Ambient System Applications Using 3D Packaging Techniques", 54th Electronic Components and Technology Conference ECTC 2004, June 1-4, 2004 Las Vegas, USA, pp 635-641.
[7] R. Tummala et al, "Microelectronics Packaging Handbook: Semiconductor Packag-ing", Kluwer Academic Publishers, January 1997.
[8] B.Majeed, et al, "Development And Thermo-Mechanical Characterisation Of 3D Folded Flex Module Used As A Technological Platform For The Realisation Of I-Seed", 3rd European Microelectronics and Packaging Symposium, June 16-18, 2004, Prague, Czech Republic.
[9] T Healy et al, "Innovative Packaging Techniques for Wearable Applications using Flexible Silicon Fibres, 54th Electronic Components and Technology Conference ECTC 2004, June 1-4, 2004 Las Vegas, USA, pp. 1216-1219.
[10] http://www.fibercomputing.net/
[11] A Applewhite. "Who knows where they are: Personal safety in the early days of Wireless", IEEE Pervasive Computing -Mobile and Ubiquitous Systems, Vol 1 (No. 3), Pages 4 – 8, Oct – Dec 2002

[12] J Barton et al, "An Inertial Measurement Unit (IMU) for an Autonomous Wireless Sensor Network", Proc. 6th Electronics Packaging Technology Conference (EPTC 2004), December 8-10, 2004, Singapore, pp. 586-589.

[13] A Mathewson et al, "The Snake-A Novel High Area Utilisation Approach for creating Integrated Circuits in Fibre Form", Irish Preliminary Patent P129447.

[14] http://www.mermoth.org/

[15] http://www.realprof.eu.com/

[16] J Barton et al, "A System For Real World Monitoring Of Prostheses And Footwear", Proc. 3rd IASTED Intern'l Conf on Biomedical Engineering, BioMED 2005, February 16-18, 2005, Innsbruck, Austria, pp. 619-623.

[17] http://www.crfprojecteu.org/menu.asp?ind=MULTIPLEYEfolder &nome=MULTIPLEYE

[18] Extrovert Gadgets (eGadgets) website, http://www.extrovert-gadgets.net

[19] http://www.tyndall.ie/research/mai-group/biot_bio_mai.html

[20] http://www.tyndall.ie/research/mai-group/biot_bio_mai.html#biomed_development

[21] http://www.tyndall.ie/research/transducers-group/bioanalyticalmicrosystemsteam.html

[22] http://www.tyndall.ie/research/mai-group/sys_int_bio_mai.html#system_real

[23] http://www.tyndall.ie/research/mai-group/device_dev_bio_mai.html

III. Standards & Interoperability

Personalised Health Management Systems
C.D. Nugent et al. (Eds.)
IOS Press, 2005

A Small Step for Science, a Big One for Commerce

Liam BIRKETT

Intellectual Property Consultant, Ireland

Abstract. The excellent work that is being performed in medical science advances is to be admired and applauded. In each case the quest is for perfection and to bring the task in hand to its final solution. Along the way there are milestones being passed that may be overlooked, as to their particular merits, because the eyes are focused all the time on the ultimate goal. The conference highlights so many areas of interest and endeavour some of which parallel, duplicate, overlap and/or compliment others.

Keywords. Intellectual property protection.

Introduction

A common cry is for more funds to facilitate the continuance of the research and development projects. In most instances these are hard to come by and so slow or limit the rate of progress. Strange as it may seem, the implementation of intellectual property matters, *from a sales and marketing perspective*, may offer a solution to many of the areas of concern.

It is worth noting that the major marketing success in the world of commerce depends greatly on branding. This is the identity that catches the attention of the consumer and is an intricate part of building loyalty. Advertising and promotion sell the benefits and explain how it is to be used but the trade mark is the vital ingredient. Once a purchaser believes in the product or service a buying pattern will be established and recommendations to others follow as a consequence. Marketing companies therefore lay great importance on the brand and the selling message.

In some instances further exclusivity can be obtained by seeking to patent the new offering. There is also now a fairly recently introduced facility known as Community Design Registration whereby the design of a product, even its ornamentation can be protected throughout the European Union, with just one application to the Office for Harmonisation in the Internal Market.

These, seemingly disparate matters, may appear at a remove from what the conference was organised to address but, in fact, can be mobilised to great effect.

During the presentations made by the experts it became clear that huge commercial opportunities were evident as asides to the central theme of the project in question. While these may be lost to the bulk of the audience, who were solely concentrating on the scientific significance of the content, the more commercially attuned participant realised the potential. Moreover, through the means of cross fertilisation, there was an opportunity for interplay between some of the advancements and discoveries being put forward by various presenters. Again, this synergy was a commercially driven one, rather than one based on the advancement of science per se.

One of the presenters was from British Telecom and laboured under the luxurious title of a futurologist. He outlined not only the capabilities that currently exist in his field, (unbeknownst to many of us), but also looked into the future. The spectacle was not only alarming but also awe-inspiring. It further provoked the concept of areas for potential collations with some of the other disciplines.

Taking this idea a stage further and considering the making of a presentation to a large marketing company the following scenario emerges. Removing the "picture if you will" approach for the more hard-nosed commercial one, a realisable product can be created. It can be branded, packaged and be capable of all forms of intellectual property protection perhaps even including patenting. It can then be put forward as a potential "ready-for-the-shelf" product.

1. An Example of Intellectual Property Protection - NAPPYHAPPY

An example of this could be the design of a nappy liner that is treated by the medical/scientific contributors to detect, when worn, health problems in babies. These may include abnormal rise in body temperature, the onset of skin problems, maybe even soiling. BT (or another Telecommunications provider) could oversee the inclusion in the weave of whatever is needed to transmit signals to a mobile phone. When problems are experienced, a signal is sent to the parent's mobile phone and action can be taken. This might entail the adult going to attend the baby or contacting the baby sitter and issuing appropriate instructions.

If the above is feasible then a brand name is created, searched to ensure that it is available for registration and an application made in the home market. That trade mark might be NAPPYHAPPY. A slogan, "Put a smile on your baby's" could also be coined; a colour combination devised to go on the packaging; a sound mark – such as – "Ma, Ma" can be registered, just like the others listed above, and a device built into the pack that emits this phrase when the pack is lifted up. All of the copy that is created around the product can enjoy copyright protection. The novel get-up and ornamentation of the packaging can avail of Registered Community Design exclusivity. It may also be possible to apply for a patent if the necessary requirements are met. Now, the product has a range of protected features that offers great attraction to the multinational. Not only is it a unique item but potential rivals are faced with an array of statutory hurdles.

While the scientific developments to achieve this stage may only be part of the way along the path to reach a more demanding goal, it has this licensing potential. This will provide attractive income but, in addition, the marketer may also be prepared to contribute to further research if offered first refusal in any new developments that ensue. In this way the research team is provided with an ongoing revenue stream plus a lump sum to meet long term objectives.

2. Consumer Benefits

By having an astute commercial awareness overseeing the scientific progress of a variety of ventures, a new dimension can be added to the current research systems. When augmented with the experience, skill and know-how to add sales appeal to a potential marketable end use a range of opportunities emerge.

The market place has an insatiable appetite for new products and services. To meet that demand novel avenues will willing be explored. If one looks to, and takes steps to promote an environment of cross fertilisation of projects, is creative and cleverly presents the outcome in a manner that has market appeal, much is to be gained.

Exciting brands are built on great consumer benefits. Major brand owners are always on the lookout for innovations that will enhance their products' appeal, such as new technologies, that will provide new, compelling benefits for consumers. Any novel insights into consumer needs are eagerly sought. A new functionality, that will create the benefit that can be promised by the brand, and enable the actual delivery of that promise, is what the marketer is after. A great insight message is something that, when heard by the targeted consumer group, is accepted by them as intrinsically right. A classic example of such an insight is the widely acknowledged fact that mothers will go to great lengths to do or buy what's best for their new baby. Proctor & Gamble's *Pampers* is the biggest selling diaper in the world. An insight in relation to a *Pampers* consumer is that they will do anything to ensure the safety and comfort of their baby. A benefit with the radically innovative *"Pampers"* mentioned above would be – now with, mobile communications, that baby need never be soiled for long. Nor will it be in more serious danger - the *Nappyhappy* will tell when it is time to change or alert them to the more serious problem. Unrivalled peace of mind!

The brand owner craves consumer loyalty. That comes from having a highly relevant benefit and how well the product delivers against that promised benefit. Great promise, ineffective functionality leaves the consumer disappointed. An ill-conceived benefit, even with great functionality - never gets anyone to try it.

3. Conclusion

Some lateral, commercial thinking is called for, which when added to that of the medical/scientific minds, can be a powerful, profitable combination. It is hoped that this small introduction to the scope of intellectual property rights, most of which are being under-utilised, will shed some light on the true potential. The simple product example should not be taken too definitively but only act as a catalyst for what can emerge if the new, suggested approach is adapted.

On the day of the conference, the writer gave the example of creating an after shave product to be marketed in Northern Ireland. The product name was STORMINT; the slogan, "a whiff of political intrigue", the symbol on the bottle was that of Stormont; the sound mark was that of the slapping of one's cheeks followed by the cry "STORMINT"; all of these plus the combination of colours on the box, were protected by registration. Everyone in attendance agreed that this product would enjoy plenty of free publicity, instant recognition and recall in the target market.

This is a hypothetical product. It does not exist yet! I rest my case.

Personalised Health Management Systems
C.D. Nugent et al. (Eds.)
IOS Press, 2005

The Efficacy of Knowledge Management for Personalised Healthcare

Rajeev K BALI[1], Ashish DWIVEDI[2] and Raouf NG NAGUIB[3]

[1]*Knowledge Management for Healthcare (KMH) research subgroup, Biomedical Computing Research Group (BIOCORE), Coventry University, United Kingdom*
[2]*Hull University Business School, University of Hull, United Kingdom*
[3]*Biomedical Computing Research Group (BIOCORE), Coventry University, United Kingdom*

Abstract. This chapter examines some of the key issues surrounding the incorporation of the Knowledge Management (KM) paradigm for personalised healthcare. We discuss the complex nature of KM, some essential concepts necessary to make personalised healthcare a reality and introduce a schematic which illustrates the efficacy of KM for personalised health.

Keywords. Clinical Knowledge Management, Personalised Healthcare, Healthcare Informatics.

Introduction

What is KM? Whom does it benefit? How is it carried out? This chapter addresses questions such as these as well as discussions as to whether it would be beneficial for healthcare stakeholders to adopt the KM paradigm so as to facilitate effective decision-making and integration in the context of healthcare delivery.

The key to the success of KM in the clinical and healthcare sectors is to achieve an effective integration of technology with human-based clinical decision-making processes. By doing so, healthcare institutions are free to disseminate acquired knowledge in a manner which ensures its availability to other healthcare stakeholders.

This is of paramount importance as healthcare and clinical management continues its growth as a global priority area. We make an analogy which demonstrates the importance and efficacy of KM for the personalised healthcare sector.

1. Clinical Knowledge Management

Advances in Information and Communication Technologies (ICT) have made it possible for healthcare institutions to transform large amounts of medical data into relevant clinical information but an average physician still spends about 25 percent of his/her time managing information and has to learn 2 million clinical specifics [1].

Biomedical literature is doubling every 19 years, a fact which further compounds the problem of information overload [2]. The notion of incorporating KM in Healthcare has been put forth as a possible solution to this problem [3,4,5].

Healthcare managers are being forced to examine costs associated with healthcare and are under increasing pressure to discover approaches that would help carry out activities better, faster and cheaper [6]. Workflow and associated Internet technologies are being seen as an instrument to cut administrative expenses.

Specifically designed Information Technology (IT) implementations such as workflow tools are being used to automate the electronic paper flow in a managed care operation, thereby cutting administrative expenses [6].

2. Evolution of IT in Healthcare

Until the early 1980s, IT solutions for healthcare used to focus on such concepts as data warehousing. The emphasis was on storage of data in an electronic medium, the prime objective of which was to allow exploitation of this data at a later point in time. As such, most of the IT applications in healthcare were built to provide support for retrospective information retrieval needs and, in some cases, to analyse the decisions undertaken. This has changed healthcare institutions' perspectives towards the concept of utility of clinical data.

Clinical data that was traditionally used in a supportive capacity for historical purposes has today become an opportunity that allows healthcare stakeholders to tackle problems before they arise.

The healthcare industry is focussed on the technology aspect of healthcare and we contend that the key to success of the healthcare sector in the twenty first century is an effective integration of technology with the human based clinical decision-making process.

One of the most challenging issues in healthcare relates to the transformation of raw clinical data into contextually relevant information. Advances in IT and telecommunications have made it possible for healthcare institutions to face the challenge of transforming large amounts of medical data into relevant clinical information [4]. This can be achieved by integrating information using workflow, context management and collaboration tools, giving healthcare a mechanism for effectively transferring the acquired knowledge, as and when required [7].

As KM deals with the tacit and contextual aspects of information, it allows an organisation to know what is important for it in particular circumstances, in the process maximising the value of that information and creating competitive advantages and wealth [8].

A KM solution would allow healthcare institutions to give clinical data context, so as to allow knowledge derivation for more effective clinical diagnoses. In the future, healthcare systems would see increased interest in knowledge recycling of the collaborative learning process acquired from previous healthcare industry practices.

This chapter puts forward the notion that this sector has been exclusively focussed on IT to meet the challenges described above and reiterates that this challenge cannot be met by an IT-led solution. The KM paradigm can enable the healthcare sector to successfully overcome the information and knowledge explosion, made possible by adopting a KM framework that is specially customised for organisations in light of their ICT implementation level [8].

3. The Efficacy of KM for Personalised Health

In order for personalised healthcare to become a reality, one needs to consider several necessary components. These include inputs from healthcare professionals, regulations and standards, perspectives from the general public and views from fashion clothing manufacturers. Given these seemingly disparate inputs, we have conceptualised them as seen in Figure 1.

3.1 The "Carpet Tile" Approach

This schematic, which we have termed the "carpet tile" approach, sees eight essential concepts ("tiles"), each one of which revolves around a central concept of KM. In our conceptualisation, we view KM as being both the central tenet as well as the "glue" which holds personalised healthcare together.

3.2 Style versus Function

Given our schematic, there is an inherent dichotomy between "looks" and functionality or form and function. As personalised healthcare involves inputs from healthcare professionals, biomedical engineers and fashion designers and manufacturers, there is a delicate balancing act between functionality and aesthetical value. This "style versus substance" quandary adds to the complexity of personalised healthcare. The solution is to encourage and engage in open and honest dialogue with all stakeholders in order that differing viewpoints can be discussed and any problems overcome.

4. Conclusions

This chapter has presented the concept of knowledge management (KM) and its efficacy for personalised healthcare. We have discussed the nature of KM and have introduced the complex relationships that exist between the multifarious inputs to the goal of personalised health and our "carpet tile" schematic makes clear this relationship.

References

[1]   A.Dwivedi, R.K.Bali, A.E.James and R.N.G.Naguib. The Efficacy of using Object Oriented Technologies to build Collaborative Applications in Healthcare and Medical Information Systems, *Proc.of the 2002 IEEE CCECE Conf. Canada*. 2002.
[2]   J.C. Wyatt, "7. Intranets," *Jnl. of The Royal Soc of Med*, **(93):10**, pp. 530-534, 2000.
[3]   AN Dwivedi, RK Bali & RNG Naguib "Organization Current Knowledge Design (OCKD): A Knowledge Management Framework for Healthcare Institutions", *Proc of the IEEE-EMBC 25th Ann Int Conf of the IEEE Eng in Med and Biol Soc (EMBS)*, 17-21 September 2003, Cancun, Mexico, 2003, 1236-1239.
[4]   SM Malone, Knowledge Management: White knight or white elephant?, *Topics in Health Information Management*. Frederick: Feb 2001. **(21):3**; 33.
[5]   S Lutz, D Chin. "Charting the landscape of healthcare in the next decade", *Managed Healthcare*. Cleveland: Nov 1999. **(9):11**; 29.
[6]   BG Latamore, "Workflow tools cut costs for high quality care," *Health Management Technology*, 1999, (20):4, 32-33.

[7]   A Dwivedi, RK Bali, AE James & RNG Naguib. "Workflow Management Systems: the Healthcare Technology of the Future *Proc of the IEEE-EMBC 25th Ann Int Conf of the IEEE Eng in Med and Biol Soc (EMBS)*, Istanbul, Turkey, 2001, 3887-3890.

[8]   RK Bali, A Dwivedi and RNG Naguib. Opportunities and Challenges for Clinical Knowledge Management", In Bali RK (2004) Clinical Knowledge Management: Opportunities and Challenges, IGP:USA, In Press.

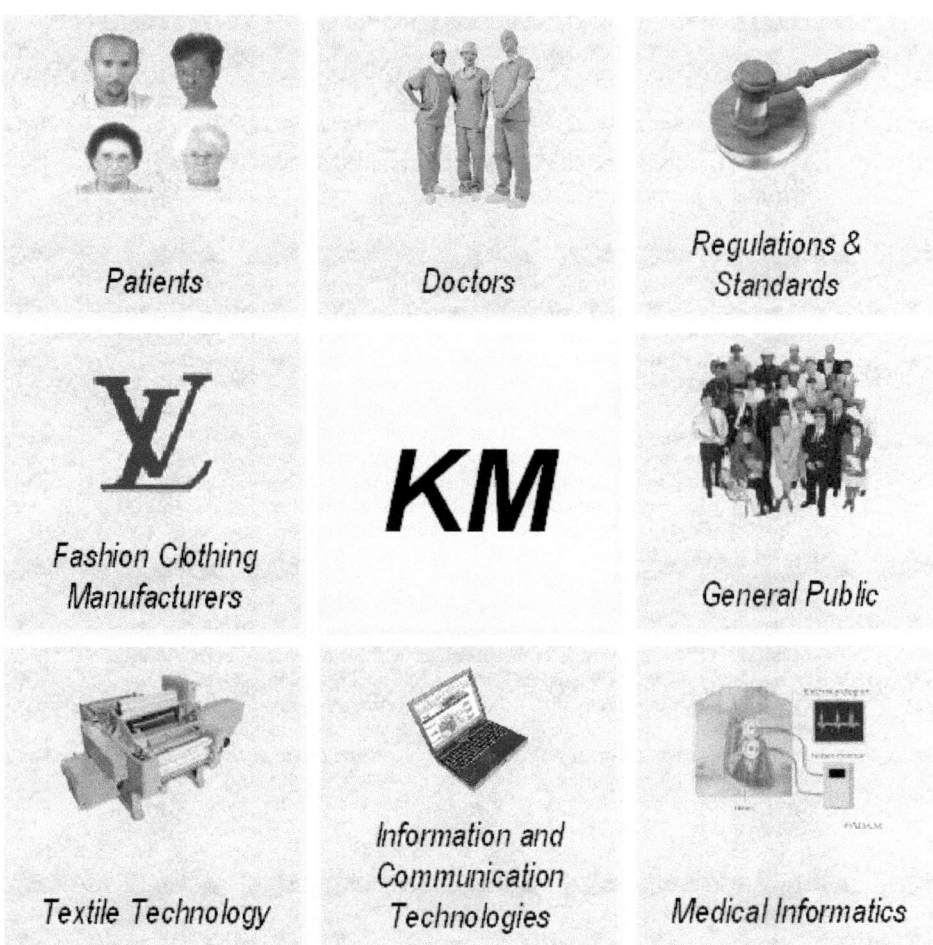

Figure 1. The "carpet tile" approach

Personalised Health Management Systems
C.D. Nugent et al. (Eds.)
IOS Press, 2005

Interoperability as a Quality Label for Portable & Wearable Health Monitoring Systems

Catherine E. CHRONAKI, Franco CHIARUGI

Institute of Computer Science, FORTH, Heraklion, Crete, Greece

Abstract. Advances in ICT promising universal access to high quality care, reduction of medical errors, and containment of health care costs, have renewed interest in electronic health records (EHR) standards and resulted in comprehensive EHR adoption programs in many European states. Health cards, and in particular the European health insurance card, present an opportunity for instant cross-border access to emergency health data including allergies, medication, even a reference ECG. At the same time, research and development in miniaturized medical devices and wearable medical sensors promise continuous health monitoring in a comfortable, flexible, and fashionable way. These trends call for the seamless integration of medical devices and intelligent wearables into an active EHR exploiting the vast information available to increase medical knowledge and establish personal wellness profiles. In a mobile connected world with empowered health consumers and fading barriers between health and healthcare, interoperability has a strong impact on consumer trust. As a result, current interoperability initiatives are extending the traditional standardization process to embrace implementation, validation, and conformance testing. In this paper, starting from the OpenECG initiative, which promotes the consistent implementation of interoperability standards in electrocardiography and supports a worldwide community with data sets, open source tools, specifications, and online conformance testing, we discuss EHR interoperability as a quality label for personalized health monitoring systems. Such a quality label would support big players and small enterprises in creating interoperable *e*Health products, while opening the way for pervasive healthcare and the take-up of the *e*Health market.

Keywords. Interoperability, Conformance testing, Health monitoring, Quality labeling, Standardization.

Introduction

Today the health sector is facing a challenge. Increasing costs in the healthcare delivery process and an aging population base call for seamless integration of diagnostic equipment, patient monitoring devices, and clinical information systems. Health cards, and in particular the European health insurance card, present an opportunity for safer mobility, better continuity of care, and cross-border sharing of medical resources. As a result, EHR standards are revisited as the means to achieve universal access to high quality care, reduction of medical errors, and containment of health care costs. At the same time, affordable portable or wearable medical devices and micro sensors increasingly support citizens in monitoring their health. Integrating the data produced by a range of medical devices in a personalized EHR for disease management and continuity of care presents an opportunity for major improvements in health care. The resulting "active" EHR may incorporate the principles of evidence-based medicine and provide feedback and alerts by analyzing the evolving health status of the individual in the context of the population at large. That is where interoperability, the ability to exchange and use meaningful information among systems, comes into play. However, interoperability is costly for manufacturers and integrators as it typically requires implementing and testing multiple communication protocols and data formats.

Several vendor/user initiatives linked to standards developing organizations (SDOs), have tried to reduce interoperability costs by organizing interoperability events such as Integrating the Healthcare Enterprise (IHE) Connectathons (www.ihe.net) or European Telecommunication Standards Institute (ETSI) Plugtests [1]. In these events that last several days each time, participating companies test their products in a controlled environment based on integration profiles. IHE has developed specialized tools -the MESA tools- to support vendors in implementing and testing integration profiles that solve real world interoperability problems. Connectathons and Plugtests facilitate standard-based integration and promote understanding, consistent implementation, and cooperative use of standards; an alternative to custom integration or auto-certification, where each vendor makes its own interoperability tests and auto-certifies its products.

However, although XML Data Synthesis (XDS) a new integration profile, addresses cross enterprise document sharing, historically the IHE has focused on hospital workflows such as patient management and scheduling of examinations. Despite the aging of the population, the prevalence of cardiovascular diseases, cancer, diabetes, etc., integration profiles for health monitoring are not fully understood or effectively implemented. Efforts in this direction are carried out by point of care standardization activities, which started back in 1983 with the IEEE Medical Information Bus. However, only recently ISO, CEN, and IEEE joined forces in the development of the IEEE 11073 family of standards. The IEEE 11073 standards provide plug-and-play interoperability for patient connected medical devices and facilitate the efficient exchange of vital signs and medical device data. They specify in detail application profiles, transport and physical layers, interworking support, application gateways, and shared concepts. In 2003, IEEE approved the core standards including the domain information model, the common nomenclature, and the basic communication profiles. Standardization of application gateways that enable communication of device-level data into EHR using HL7 V2.5 together with elements of ISO/IEEE 11073 is also underway. Nevertheless, standards dealing with plug-interoperability of medical devices into an active EHR are still nascent. Intense collaboration is necessary to create, test, validate, and adopt gateways for effective alarm management and health monitoring.

Regional health information networks and rising demands for interoperability in *e*Health were driving forces behind OpenECG, which was funded by the EU (2002-2004) to promote standards and open data formats in electrocardiography. OpenECG managed to reduce interoperability costs with the first online conformance testing service for ECG records in the Standard Communications Protocol (SCP)-ECG standard. The success of the OpenECG initiative indicates that community effort, open source, and high quality services have a positive impact on the adoption of interoperability standards.

In the rest of the chapter we outline the objectives, activities, and results of the OpenECG project (section 1) and we analyze the conformance testing service developed for the SCP-ECG standard (section 2) to illustrate a practical example of how interoperability support can be rewarded by the market as a quality label. Then, we move to section 3 to discuss EHR interoperability as a quality label for health monitoring and intelligent textiles. Section 4 presents our conclusions.

1. Data Sets, Specifications and Open Source Components

Standards Development Organisations (SDOs) are dedicated to the preparation of standards with voluntarily involvement of major stakeholders. Several times it happens that a well-written standard is not implemented by manufacturers and there are at least three possible reasons for that. First, manufacturers are not aware of the existence of standards. This was true in the past where each medical device needed to be validated in different countries where different standards could apply. Today standards can be used to verify all over Europe that essential requirements for patient safety are met and manufacturers should be very interested in being up-to-date with the existing standards. Indeed, interoperability is increasingly recognized as an aspect of patient safety due to its potential impact on quality care, reduction of errors, and effective utilization of knowledge. Second, manufacturers are not willing to adopt an open protocol/format, but they are prepared to use a proprietary closed solution. Since standards start to be strongly required in procurements, this position can no longer be maintained. Third, manufacturers claim (mainly Small and Medium-sized Enterprises) that they cannot afford a large investment for the implementation of a very complex standard. Thus, standards need to be published with supporting tools, services, and software for easy implementation and interoperability support.

The OpenECG project started in June 2002. Driving forces were patient mobility, regional networks, continuity of care, and the vision of the life-long EHR [2]. At that time, virtually all cardiology examinations involving measurements of vital signs required the software suite of the specific manufacturer to collect, store, and analyze the data. Changing the device would imply losing all previous data or launching a costly data migration effort. Furthermore, in a regional network where the list of medical devices is open-ended, plug-interoperability is an integrator's dream. The best way to realize this dream is by establishing a community to raise awareness, share expertise, and promote best practice in implementation. OpenECG did exactly that, and moreover it focused its efforts on supporting the consistent implementation of standards and alleviating interoperability problems by providing feedback to SDOs on the limitations of existing standards. The starting point was the typical 12 lead resting ECG. The OpenECG project provided rich support for ECG interoperability: (a) links to specifications, (b) tutorials, (c) help desk to answer to specific questions, (d) data sets of ideal and real implementations of the SCP-ECG standard, (e) ECG data and viewers in other formats (Medical waveform Format Encoding Rules and Health Level 7 Annotated ECG), (f) format converters (SCP-ECG to DICOM waveform sup. 30), (g) Open Source Software Tools Repository with source code of SCP-ECG parsers, viewers, and other tools.

OpenECG is committed to open software for viewing, measuring, and analyzing the ECG, the most common non-invasive examination for those at risk or living with heart disease. In fact, a strongly supported viewpoint within the OpenECG community is that the poor diffusion of standards is partly due to the lack of public software. To cope with this problem, OpenECG decided to adopt and promote the "open-source/free-software" strategy in software development and use. Free software seems to be a natural choice when dissemination of results and co-operation is the key for increasing knowledge and for exchanging/evaluating new products and ideas. Thus, the OpenECG SW Tools Repository came up as an annotated collection of open source and shareware tools for viewing, processing, and translation of ECGs. Furthermore, a programming contest was organized to stimulate the creation of tools necessary to integrate digital ECGs into the healthcare workflows. It was launched in January 2003 and gave out prizes of 10000 Euro in total to the best open source tools for ECG viewing, analyzing, or format conversion. These tools, now available in the OpenECG SW Tools repository together with tools contributed by members, show the way from "paper" standards towards interoperability standards that actually work. Although, today most ECGs world-wide are diagnosed on paper, the tools of the repository uncouple ECG viewing, analysis, diagnosis, and storage from specific device models. Now the medical community has to take the lead and establish guidelines for over-reading of ECGs and other vital signs.

The OpenECG portal (www.openecg.net) is a valuable resource for open ECGs data formats. Today, there are several data formats for digital ECGs characterized by various levels of adoption. Besides raw data, there is SCP-ECG, the European interchange format, FEF a data format associated with the VITAL standard (ISO/CEN/IEEE 11073) for vital signs measurements, MFER a Japanese format able to represent any time series of health data, and MSD a recent data format addressing the particular needs of micro sensors [3]. Furthermore, following the requirement for full disclosure of data collected in the course of clinical trials, the FDA commissioned the development of the Annotated ECG format, which has been endorsed by HL7. Making sense of all the different formats, as well as testing and quality assurance of data sets, require the support of experts. This is the role assumed by the OpenECG network. So far, the OpenECG community has been effective in assuring the quality of data sets from ECG vendors, even spotting missing information or minor discrepancies.

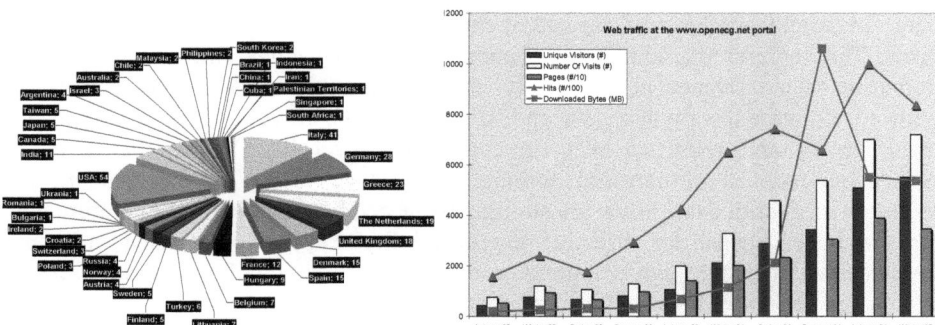

Figure 1: The OpenECG community is steadily growing (340 members in 44 countries). Traffic in the www.openecg.net portal is also rising, while Google returns more and more links to OpenECG.

The OpenECG community has been steadily growing to reach 340 members (235 from Europe) in 44 countries in January 2005. Members are primarily from academic institutes (42%), the industry (40%), and healthcare organizations (16%). Member applications arrive regularly at a frequency of 2-3 per week. Most of these applications come from the industry, the academia, and increasingly from IT personnel working for healthcare organizations. Each member is individually contacted to provide a statement of purpose for joining the OpenECG community. At the same time, traffic on the OpenECG portal since its launching in autumn 2002, has increased 10-fold (Fig.1). Moreover, a dramatic increase in downloads starting from summer 2004, underlines the role of the portal as a resource for software, sample data, and technical documentation.

2. Conformance Testing for Interoperability: The Case of SCP-ECG

The aim of OpenECG is to achieve interoperability through stable and robust standards that have been extensively validated in practice. Since September 2003, OpenECG tests the conformance of ECG records and devices against the Standard Communications Protocol for Electrocardiography (SCP-ECG, EN 1064:1994; 2002). SCP-ECG is a published standard, allowing connectivity between ECG instruments and host systems. With SCP-ECG, compatible systems can transmit, store, and receive ECGs with full waveform fidelity. Although SCP-ECG is a comprehensive standard, it has not been adopted to the degree expected. It was first published in 1994 and it covers an interchange format and a limited number of messages for the acquisition, transfer, and storage of 12-lead ECGs. An SCP-ECG record comprises several sections including Code Redundancy Check (CRC) for the whole record and for each section. Sections include demographics (section 1), rhythm data (section 6), measurements (section 7), and diagnostic statements (section 8). The standard also specifies methods for rhythm data compression that may reduce the size of the SCP-ECG file tenfold down to about 10 Kbytes; a convenient size for health cards and micro sensors.

The SCP-ECG standard specifies four compliance levels: I, II, III, IV. Compliance level I requires the transmission or storage in an SCP-ECG file of demographics, measurements, and diagnostic statements (sections 0, 1, 7, 8). The purpose of this conformance level is to facilitate communication of the diagnostic report without attaching the actual rhythm data. In compliance level II, rhythm data is included. This requires also sections 2, 3, 6 to include Huffman tables, lead definition, and rhythm data. In compliance level III, instead of rhythm data, manufacturers include reference beats. This requires the addition of sections 2, 3, 5 to include Huffman tables, lead definition, and reference beats. Finally, in compliance level IV, manufacturers are allowed to introduce rhythm data and reference beats. Rhythm data in compliance levels II, IV and reference beats in compliance level III, IV may be stored in redundancy-reduced compressed format. Compliance levels II, IV demand the inclusion of rhythm data, which are strongly requested by cardiologists. Therefore they are the better choice for effective interoperability. On the other hand, a proper implementation of the high compression method is quite complex and conformance testing can be a lot of help.

OpenECG members may test the conformance of ECG devices and ECG records to the SCP-ECG standard. Conformance testing assists integrators and manufacturers, who consider endorsement by OpenECG a quality label for their products. Before OpenECG, the only option available was auto-certification, i.e., self-declaration of conformance to standards or interoperability with equipment of certain vendors.

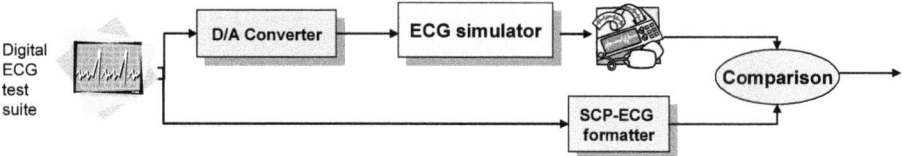

Figure 2: The process of ECG device Testing.

ECG Device testing is available offline. The vendor or user needs to provide a statement of compliance, the SCP-ECG implementation document, and the device itself, accompanied by appropriate documentation of the communication protocol and software drivers for interconnectivity. The low level details of the communication protocol managed by a driver are beyond the scope of conformance testing. It is the driver that has to be able to retrieve the ECG data recording into a "claimed" SCP-ECG record. This record is accessible to the OpenECG conformance testing service through the file system or a DBMS with disclosed structure. An analog ECG data set is used to test the conformance of ECG devices to the SCP-ECG standard. Each ECG signal is fed into the device under test through a simulator. Then, the recorded ECG records are compared to the original input data in the SCP-ECG format (see Fig. 2).

Any authenticated OpenECG member may submit an SCP-ECG file for automatic online conformance testing. Conformance testing for SCP-ECG files comprises detailed checking of the content and format of the data sections. After about 400 conformity tests based on the specifications of SCP-ECG v1.0 and v1.3, a report is automatically produced. The report includes warning messages that refer to recommendations that are not met and errors that indicate failure in meeting mandatory requirements of the SCP-ECG standard.

Conformance tests are realized using the content and format checker [4]. The content checker reads the ECG file assuming it is written in the SCP-ECG standard and generates an output file, which contains header information including the name and size of the SCP-ECG file, the CRC code, and the SCP-ECG keyword. If the SCP-ECG record is compressed, it also includes Huffman tables, ECG lead definition, QRS locations, and reference beats if the compliance level is III or IV. If compliance level is II or IV, it includes Rhythm data. It may also report, if present, global measurements, lead measurements, and diagnostic statements. The format checker examines compliance of sections 0 to 6 to the ECG record with format specifications of SCP-ECG standard performing global format tests, common tests, and section dependent tests. Global format tests include testing of global CRC, record length, and presence of mandatory SCP-ECG sections. Common tests include testing of even section length, local CRC, and section length for all sections present. Section dependent tests apply only to sections 0...6 in the current version of the format checker, but other sections may be included in the future. When conformance testing is successful, an OpenECG certificate is awarded describing the conditions of the tests.

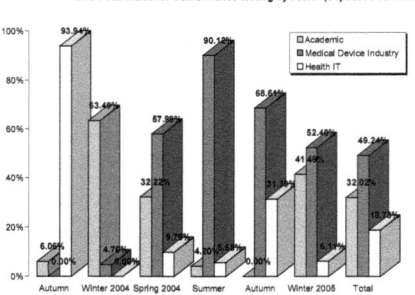

Figure 3: There is consistent interest of the industry in online conformance testing.

The online conformance testing service has been used 327 times by 22 members of the OpenECG community, since September 2003. Approximately 6% of the members use the service on a regular basis. They come from the industry (9), the academia (8), and IT departments in major hospitals (5). Up to January 2005, online conformance testing has assisted 3 companies in developing an SCP-ECG implementation, while 2 hospital IT departments realized an interoperable solution with ECG machines from different vendors. Fig. 3 shows a steadily increasing interest of the industry in using online conformance testing. Online conformance testing serves a global community; members that regularly use the service come from Austria, Finland, France, Germany, Italy, Japan, the Netherlands, Rumania, Spain, Taiwan, Turkey, UK, and USA.

The ECG records submitted to the conformance testing service are stored anonymized in a database available online to members of the OpenECG network. Periodic review of the submitted ECGs and conformance testing results assists us not only in recognizing common implementation errors, but also in assuring the quality of the testing tools. Based on comments from the community the testing tools have already been revised once. As the members keep on using the service, the quality and accuracy of the service further improve. Currently, we are in the process of designing and implementing a web service that will make the testing tools available to members not only over the web, but also as part of their software. This development will increase the robustness of ECG viewing and archiving software as it will alert in cases that an acquired ECG does not conform to the levels of quality demanded by SCP-ECG.

Online conformance testing in the portal turns out to be a key to substantial improvement in the adoption of the standard and the level of interoperability attained in practice. The trust that members have rested on the collective experience of the OpenECG community is a driving force and a paradigm to follow for standardization activities realizing plug-interoperability of medical devices into an active EHR.

3. Interoperability as a Quality Label

Frequently for the sake of manufacturer endorsement, standards include optional parameters like the manufacturer-specific sections and additional tags in section 1 of the SCP-ECG standard. That may be an obstacle to interoperability. Currently, within CEN TC251/WGIV there is a motion to reduce the compliance levels of SCP-ECG to simplify the standard and increase its usability in achieving interoperability. Indeed, very few standards are robust and adequately supported in implementation to realize true interoperability. Even when two vendors claim conformance to the same standard, due to allowable options in the standard, there is no guarantee that their products will interoperate. Lack of rigorous conformance testing and certification procedures for interoperability leaves manufacturers with auto-certification as the only option.

With standardization there is always the issue of how much regulation should be advocated, since frequently overregulation hampers innovation [5]. On the other hand, there is no doubt that lack of interoperability is limiting innovation. In case of the ECG, which is considered as personal as a fingerprint, a cardiologist following the ECG of a patient overtime can better appreciate variations of the physiological signal or monitor the individual's heart disease. However, at a time when web services can provide access to online processing and serial comparison of ECGs, there is no single accepted format for storage of ECGs as waveforms in the EHR. Plug-interoperability among devices and EHRs would facilitate the creation of databases to assess inter/intra subject variability and specify alarm levels in the context of individualized health monitoring [6]. In this way, the gap would narrow between the data collected at the point of care and the actual knowledge that can be obtained to deliver effective healthcare.

The medical device sector is conservative and over-regulated. Therefore, partly to protect their market share and partly to reduce development costs, manufacturers are very hesitant towards implementing standards. They prefer robust vertical applications of limited functionality that address essential regulatory requirements for patient safety and short-term user needs. Interoperability standards claim to provide solutions for integrated care, but it is not quite so. In its report on achieving interoperability the CEN/ISSS *e*Health focus group notes that official standards are frequently not well-known and not used, while some of them are even conflicting. Furthermore, there is a lack of guidance on where and how to use standards. The main recommendation of the report is to create an interoperability platform that will encourage and promote interoperability of systems based on standards within an environment for research, testing, evaluation, and certification [7].

To promote consumer trust, we propose that the industry, supported by medical professionals and patient organizations, should create a quality label along the lines of Bluetooth (www.bluetooth.com). Bluetooth is a private trade association that provides a forum for companies to work together using short-range wireless technologies. All members of the Bluetooth SIG have permission to use Bluetooth wireless technology in their products and services. In the same way, companies involved in health monitoring should join forces to realize plug-interoperability of their products to active personalized EHRs. Data formats, nomenclature and a domain model would be a shared resource, while an open platform would facilitate managing the shared context, i.e. who is the patient, what is his/her normal range of measurements, and so on.

4. Conclusions

The integration of low-cost interoperable health monitoring devices for telemedicine and personal health management holds high potential for the *e*Health market, assuming interoperability issues are effectively resolved. The success of OpenECG suggests that a quality label associated with plug-interoperability of medical devices to active EHR systems would establish consumer trust on *e*Health and promote pervasive health care in the next generation working and living environments.

Acknowledgements

OpenECG was funded under EU contract IST-2001-377111. The authors would like to thank Chr. Zywietz, F. Conforti, A. Macerata, M. Bruun-Rasmussen, PJ. Lees, I. Johansen, H. Voss, J. Perez, R. Ruiz, & the OpenECG community who make it happen.

References

[1]   S. Mooseley, S. Randall, A. Wiles, In Pursuit of Interoperability, *J of IT Standards & Standardization Research*, **2**(2), 34-38, July-Dec 2004.
[2]   P.J. Lees, C.E. Chronaki, F. Chiarugi, Standards and Interoperability in Digital Electrocardiography. The OpenECG Project, *Hellenic Journal of Cardiology*, **45**:364-369, 2004.
[3]   Proceedings of the *2nd OpenECG workshop*: "Integration of the ECG into the EHR & Interoperability of ECG device systems: where we are – where we are going..", Berlin 1-4 April 2004.
[4]   Chr. Zywietz, R. Fischer, "Integrated Content and Format Checking for Processing of SCP ECG Records", In Murray A(ed): *Computers in Cardiology* 2004; **31** *(In press)*
[5]   G. Swan, The economics of standardization, Manchester Business School, *Final report for standards and technical regulations directorate*, December 2000
[6]   Chr. Zywietz, Communication and Interoperability for Serial Comparison in Continuous Health Care – the new Challenges, In *Wearable eHealth Systems for Personalized Health Management*, A. Lymberis and D. de Rossi, editors, p. 172-180, IOS Press, 2004
[7]   CEN/ISSS eHealth Standardization Focus Group, http://www.centc251.org/ehealthfocusgroup.htm

Personalised Health Management Systems
C.D. Nugent et al. (Eds.)
IOS Press, 2005

Software Process Improvement for the Medical Industry

Fergal McCAFFERY[1], Peter DONNELLY[2], Donald McFALL[1] and
Frederick George WILKIE[1]
[1]*Centre for Software Process Technologies, University of Ulster,
Northern Ireland.*
[2]*IQ Solutions, Castlewellan, Northern Ireland.*

Abstract. This chapter describes a software process improvement framework, structured to ensure regulatory compliance for the software developed in medical devices. Software is becoming an increasingly important aspect of medical devices and medical device regulation. Medical devices can only be marketed if compliance and approval from the appropriate regulatory bodies of the Food and Drug Administration (US requirement), and the European Commission under its Medical Device Directives (CE marking requirement) is achieved.

Keywords: Software Process Improvement, Process assessment, Process areas, Process Capability, 3CMMI® , Regulatory compliance.

Introduction

Of increased interest to medical device companies, particularly small businesses, is to enhance their software development processes beyond the sole need to ensure regulatory compliance, into an environment that integrates compliance, best practice and process improvement. The software framework introduced in this chapter will address an opportunity to integrate the regulatory issues and process improvement mechanisms in order to improve the quality of software produced by medical device companies. Integrated into the design process of medical devices, is a requirement for the production and maintenance of a device technical file, incorporating a design history file. Design history illustrates the well documented, defined and controlled processes and outputs, undertaken in the development of medical devices and for our particular consideration with this framework - the software components.

---

[3] "CMMI is registered in the U.S. Patent and Trademark Office by Carnegie Mellon University"

1. Background

A recent survey performed by IQ Solutions with the medical device companies in Northern Ireland (NI) has revealed that the software development process has been predominately based on the need to comply with the US Food and Drug Administration (FDA) [1] and European Medical Device Directives (MDD) [2] regulations. The software lifecycle process itself has not been of primary focus, only that the elements are in place that satisfy the regulatory requirements.

It is believed that a Software Process Improvement (SPI) exercise would greatly enhance the design control procedures currently being implemented in company quality systems [3]. The major rationale for the software framework is to improve software quality and reduce time to market. Quality software is defined as software that meets its functional and non-functional requirements without lengthy rework, including regulatory compliance, without any inconsistencies. Reducing time to market is often based on continuous improvement of processes implemented for the design, development and manufacture of medical devices and products.

2. SPI framework

The Centre for Software Process Technologies (CSPT) is a research and knowledge transfer group funded jointly by the University of Ulster and a Northern Ireland governmental organisation charged with the economic development of this geographical region. The CSPT is tasked with motivating and supporting a culture of software process improvement within the NI software industry. The CSPT and IQ Solutions are developing a software process improvement framework for the medical device sector that integrates existing regulatory requirements for the control of the design, development, maintenance and support of software, with a software process improvement mechanism that will improve quality.

The approach for delivering the SPI framework is to establish a Medical Device Software Process Improvement (MeDeSPI) model (implemented as illustrated in Figure 1) that addresses the specific software development requirements from relevant regulatory bodies, standards, customer expectations, and integrates those constraints with an existing SPI framework. The MeDeSPI model identifies relevant components of the continuous version of the Capability Maturity Model Integration (CMMI®) for Software Engineering [4]. The MeDeSPI model will be flexible in that relevant elements of the model may be adopted as required to provide the most significant benefit to the business.

The major process improvement frameworks that currently exist, namely ISO/IEC15004 [5] and CMMI®, do not address the regulatory requirements of the medical device industry. The US Food and Drug Administration (FDA) and the European Medical Device Directives (MDD) are the regulatory standards that control the design, development, manufacturing and support of products within the medical device industry.

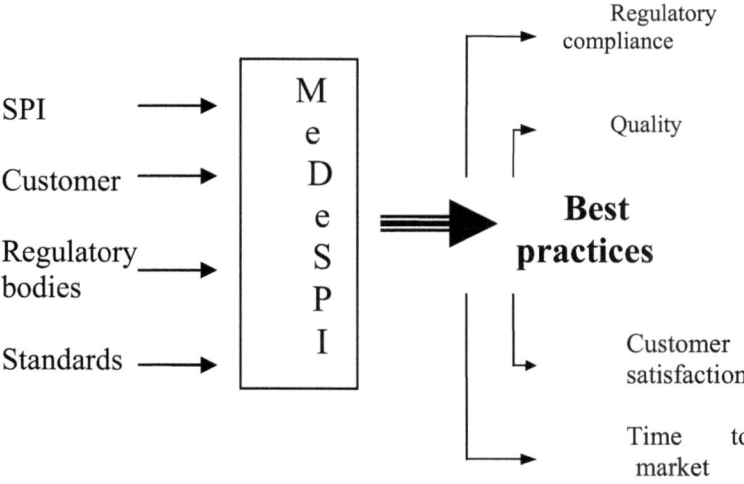

Figure 1. Medical Device Software Process Improvement (MedeSPI) model.

3. Project Outline

In order to deliver an endorsed framework it was essential that a steering group was formed with members from various medical device companies and a notified body with experience in auditing medical device companies. The involvement of medical device companies also adds an ownership element to the model and should improve its acceptance and implementation within each company. The software development model will cover the complete lifecycle. No restriction will be made on the development lifecycle processes undertaken by individual companies, although it is understood that companies within the medical device sector typically implement this V-Model. The model will be expanded to incorporate applicable aspects CMMI® in addition to checking that all applicable standards and regulations are adhered to in a seamless manner and are focused upon software process improvement.

The MeDeSPI model will also ensure that developed, reused or off-the-shelf [6] software satisfies functional, operational and regulatory requirements throughout the software development lifecycle. As each stage of the lifecycle can be performed using various methodologies and project management processes, the model will be flexible to support the implementation and integration of preferred methodologies into the framework.

The framework will also provide a software development roadmap, which complies with the regulatory guidance criteria, while introducing best practice techniques and methodologies that can be selected as required. For example a risk management process can adopt a Failure Mode and Effects Analysis (FMEA) method of identifying, mitigating and tracking risk and hazard issues. Also the continuous management of verification and validation testing can be controlled and planned under a structured test process improvement model.

4. Process Assessment

The MeDeSPI model will provide a structured approach for appraisal that may be used by organisations involved in the development, maintenance and support of software with the following purposes:

- Understanding the state of a company's own processes for process improvement;
- Determining the capability of a company's own processes for a particular contract;
- Determining the capability of another organisation's processes for a particular contract.

Process assessment is an integral part of software process improvement and provides a way to measure the capability of selected processes in an organisation against a target capability profile. Analysis of the assessment results enables companies to prioritise which processes should be improved in order to increase their effectiveness in achieving their business goals. The assessment results will also indicate the risks involved in undergoing a project using the assessed processes. This enables determination of how effective they are in achieving their goals, and to identify significant causes of poor quality, or overruns in time or cost. These provide the criteria to prioritise process improvements.

The process assessment (MeDeSPI) model is composed of two main components:

- Process areas;
- Capability scale.

Section 4.1 lists the process areas that are deemed applicable to the medical device industry. Section 4.2 details the capability scale against which each process is measured. The capability scale is based upon CMMI® capability scales. Section 4.3 outlines the activities performed in an assessment.

4.1. Process Areas

The assessment method will provide a means of assessing software engineering capability in twelve areas that have been defined by the FDA [7] as:

1. Level of Concern;
2. Software Description;
3. Device Hazard and Risk Analysis;
4. Software Requirements Specification;
5. Architecture Design;
6. Design Specifications;
7. Requirements Traceability Analysis;
8. Development;
9. Validation, Verification and Testing [8];
10. Revision Level History;
11. Unresolved Anomalies;
12. Release Version Number.

To ensure compliance whilst also achieving software process improvement the following twelve CMMI® software process areas have been deemed appropriate for the medical device industry as a mapping can be made from these process areas to the twelve areas listed above:

1. Project Planning;
2. Project Monitoring & Control;
3. Supplier Agreement Management;
4. Risk Management;
5. Requirements Management;
6. Requirements Development;
7. Technical Solution;
8. Product Integration;
9. Verification;
10. Validation;
11. Configuration Management;
12. Process and Product Quality Assurance.

The mappings between the FDA regulatory guidelines and the CMMI® process areas listed above then produce twelve MeDeSPI process areas which retain the CMMI® process area names listed above. The MeDeSPI assessment model will therefore be composed of these twelve process areas. Each of the MeDeSPI process areas will then be composed of a number of goals and practices. Goals and practices may be either generic (relating to the entire organisation) or specific (relating to the current process area). MeDeSPI investigates what parts of the CMMI® process areas are required to satisfy FDA regulations, but also investigates the possibility of extending the CMMI® process areas with additional goals and practices that are outside the remit of CMMI®, but are required in order to satisfy FDA regulations. The composition of the MeDeSPI model is illustrated in Figure 2.

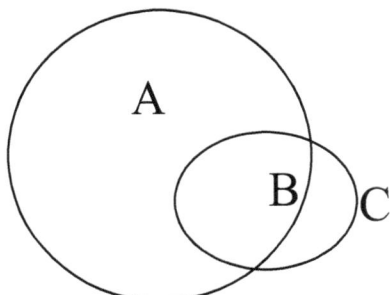

A-   CMMI® Practices that are not mandatory for FDA compliance.
B-   CMMI® Practices that are required for FDA compliance.
C-   Non- CMMI® Practices that are required for FDA compliance.

Figure 2. Composition of the MeDeSPI model.

4.2. Capability Scale Section

The MeDeSPI model will help companies to measure their organisational capability and to track progression and achievements in each of the twelve process areas and against process capability levels. The MeDeSPI assessment model has adopted the following capability levels:

- **Level 0** – Companies must demonstrate that a process area satisfies the goals and performs the practices required to achieve FDA regulatory compliance. This will involve performing some practices which the CMMI® views as generic, although not to the extent of fulfilling any generic goals;
- **Level 1** - Companies must demonstrate that a process area satisfies level 0 and the CMMI® capability level 1 goal of performing the CMMI® base practices;
- **Level 2** – Companies must demonstrate that a process area satisfies level 1 and additionally performs CMMI® Advanced Practices, as well as the CMMI® capability level 2 generic goal of Institutionalising a Managed Process;
- **Level 3** - Companies must demonstrate that a process area satisfies level 2 and additionally the CMMI® Generic Goal to Institutionalise a Defined Process (CMMI® Generic Goal 3);
- **Level 4** – Companies must demonstrate that a process area satisfies level 3 and additionally the CMMI® Generic Goal to Institutionalise a Quantitatively Managed Process (CMMI® Generic Goal 4);
- **Level 5** - Companies must demonstrate that a process area satisfies level 4 and additionally the CMMI® Generic Goal to Institutionalise an Optimising Process (CMMI® Generic Goal 5).

The assessment model will help companies to measure their organisational capability and to track progression and achievements in each of the twelve process areas.

4.3. Assessment Method Activities

To perform a MeDeSPI assessment the following activities will have to be performed:

- Request for process assessment;
- Planning the assessment schedule;
- Briefing the company in relation to the assessment;
- Performing the assessment and collecting information;
- Analysing and validating the information collected;
- Providing a rating for the process area;
- Reporting and inputs to the risk management process.

Each process area included in the assessment will be appraised on the basis of available evidence. The evidence may be gathered using interview, inspecting organisational documents or analysing metrics. The information collected for each process area will be compared against assessment objectives and scope for that process area. Information that supports a particular process rating will be recorded and maintained as evidence to substantiate the ratings and to verify compliance with the requirements.

The assessment method activities include a last important step "Reporting and providing inputs to the risk management process". The risk management process area is both a process area and the final step of the assessment activities, as it is important that risk management is assigned a separate process area and that issues found in other process areas are also reported into the risk management process. This is particularly important to software developed or implemented in the medical device industry, as it is necessary to implement a risk management strategy throughout development. The risk management guidelines within the framework will acknowledge and endorse the ISO14971:2000 standard for "Application of Risk Management to Medical Devices".

5. Improving Software Process Area Through Using the MeDeSPI Model

Software process improvement is a continuous process that an organisation follows in a cyclic improvement path of performing an assessment, implementing the recommendations from the assessment to achieve improvement, and then starting the cycle again by reassessing to check for improvement. Improvement will be achieved by following this path and adopting specific improvement measures such as the introduction of new or changed practices into established processes and removing inefficient practices. An important step within the software process improvement cycle is the gathering of information. This information is required to establish the current state and subsequently to confirm the improvements by comparing the initial process assessment results with the re-assessment results gathered after the implementation of the improvements.

6. Conclusion

Of particular importance to medical device companies is the need to develop medical devices in full compliance with the appropriate regulatory bodies that govern the sale and marketing of medical devices throughout the world. The key business goals of cost effective development and speed to market, are fundamental factors for all companies, but for small new-start companies this is critical. The studies and assessment of the Northern Ireland medical device industry illustrates that the MeDeSPI model as proposed in this chapter will provide a huge benefit to participating companies as business goals and regulatory compliance may both be achieved. The MeDeSPI model is still undergoing development.

Acknowledgements

The Centre for Software Process Technologies at the University of Ulster is supported by the EU Programme For Peace And Reconciliation in Northern Ireland and The Border Region Of Ireland (PEACE II).

References

[1]   FDA Regulations. "Code of Federal Regulations 21 CFR Part 820." June 1997.
[2]   European Council, "Council Directive 93/42/EEC Concerning Medical Devices", 14 June 1993.
[3]   F. Mc Caffery , P. Donnelly, A. Dorling & F.G. Wilkie. (Apr 2004) "A Software Process Development, Assessment and Improvement Framework for the Medical Device Industry", Proceedings of Fourth

International SPICE Conference on Process Assessment and Improvement, Lisbon, Portugal, 28-29 April 2004, SPICE User Group (Lisbon, Portugal), ISBN 972-9071-73-X, Pages 100-109.

[4]   Capability Maturity Model® Integration (CMMI[SM]) for Software Engineering (CMMI-SW, V1.1, Version 1.1, August 2002).

[5]   ISO/IEC TR 15504:1998(E), Information Technology – Software Process Assessment, Parts 1-9, Type 2 Technical report.

[6]   FDA/CDRH Guidance Document. "Guidance for Off-the-Shelf Software Use in Medical Devices." September 1999.

[7]   FDA/CDRH Guidance Document. "Guidance for the Content of Premarket Submissions for Software Contained in Medical Devices." May 1998.

[8]   FDA/CDRH Guidance Document. "General Principles of Software Validation." June 1997.

Personalised Health Management Systems
C.D. Nugent et al. (Eds.)
IOS Press, 2005

Interoperability - a Key Infrastructure Requirement for Personalised Health Services

Thomas NORGALL

Fraunhofer IIS
Am Wolfsmantel 33, D-91058 Erlangen,
http://www.iis.fraunhofer.de/

Abstract. Functional and semantic interoperability requirements for ubiquitous personalised health services reach beyond current concepts of health information integration among professional stakeholders and related Electronic Patient Records ("eHealth"): Future health telematics infrastructures have particularly to maintain semantic interoperability among systems using different coding schemes and terminologies and to include home, personal and mobile systems.

Keywords. Functional and semantic interoperability, e-Health, health telematics, communication standards, Body Area Network, micro-systems, Personal Health.

Introduction: Functional and Semantic Interoperability for e-Health

Health information integration ("eHealth") implies interoperability among all clinical and healthcare-related institutions and stakeholders (Figure 1). Electronic Health Records (EHR) comprise relevant demographic, diagnostic and therapeutic information. It is generated, stored and used by different stakeholders at different places and different points in time. Nevertheless, it may be required and processed simultaneously in a specific situation during a patient's treatment. Other typical eHealth applications like e-letter, e-consultation or e-prescription involve multiple stakeholders, partly on an ad-hoc basis: hospitals, general practitioners and specialists, pharmacies, labs and care service providers, insurance companies etc. To make all this happen, "health telematics" infrastructure – being currently developed or introduced in all industrialised countries – has to provide for adequate functional and semantic interoperability.

The IEEE Standard Computer Dictionary [1] defines interoperability as *"the ability of two or more systems or components to exchange information and to use the information that has been exchanged"*. Interoperability may comprise capabilities of systems or components to *exchange information* ("functional interoperability", e.g. by shared architectures, protocols, frameworks) and to *use the information that has been exchanged* ("semantic interoperability", e.g. by terminology and coding schemes) without further need for user interaction. Functional interoperability is a prerequisite for semantic interoperability.

Communication standards are essential for interoperability of communicating systems and integration of information. Communication architectures, interfaces, transmission protocols and codes tend to be unnecessarily limited to specific components, applications, manufacturers or domains, resulting in barriers, efforts and costs when exchanging information or even just replacing components. Motivated by this situation, groups of professionals from different clinical areas started work on standardisation of medical data exchange and communication. Their objective was primarily to improve the situation in their particular environments. Resulting standards established in specific domains are generally based on incompatible concepts reflecting not only typical domain-specific requirements and conceptual paradigms, but also their development history. However, these originally clinical standards have to be utilised for "eHealth".

1. Interoperability Domains, Standards and Concepts

1.1. From Clinical "Information Islands" to Interoperability

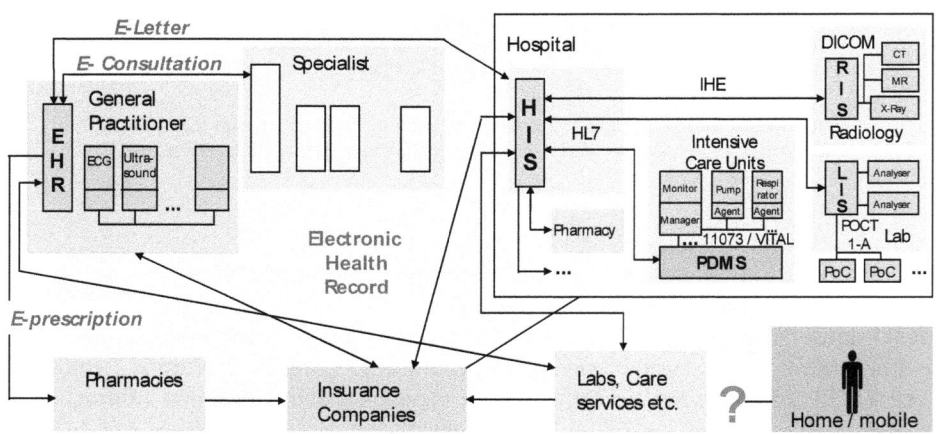

Figure 1. Typical "eHealth" stakeholders, systems, interaction and integration paths.

Hospitals were the first institutions that utilised computers for healthcare applications. They are usually operating a data processing system for patient administration and basic patient data (demographics, diagnoses and procedures), mostly referred to as Hospital Information System (HIS). HIS architecture has dramatically changed over the past 30 years. Today a network of distributed computers systems is used, each system specialised for domain-specific applications. Examples are lab systems for order/sample/result administration and quality control, Radiology Information System (RIS) and/or Picture Archiving and Communications System (PACS) in radiology departments, intensive care units (ICU) with patient data management (documentation) systems, etc. (Figure 1). A central core system handles basic patient data and keeps track of patient treatment across different departments. It builds up a basic patient record including links to patient-related information stored by departmental systems. In the mid-80s a group of US system vendors and users formed a consortium called "Health Level 7" (HL7) [2] with reference to the application layer in the ISO/OSI reference model. They started work on the standardisation of message structures (abstract message definition), the representation of messages for transmission (encoding rules) and triggering events (message triggers). Version 2.x series of HL7 standards was most successful and is widely used for HIS communication as well as interfacing between hospitals, insurance companies and public health organisations. Ambiguities in specifications and difficult handling of options due to a complete lack of formal models motivated the ongoing development of object-model-based XML-encoded HL7 Version 3.

In 1993 the American College of Radiology (ACR) and the National Electrical Manufacturers Association (NEMA) published the first version of their standard to be called "Digital Imaging and Communications in Medicine" (DICOM) [3]. It specified a network protocol utilising TCP/IP, service classes extending the simple transfer of data and an identification mechanism for information objects. DICOM Information Objects are not only images but also patients, studies, reports, etc. DICOM has a multi-part structure to facilitate extensions of the Standard. With its supplements, DICOM specifies the communication of digital images from different modalities like computer tomographs (CT), magnetic resonance tomographs (MR) etc. to diagnostic workstations, picture archiving and communication systems (PACS) etc. and also facilitates interfacing with clinical information systems.

The "Point-of-Care Connectivity Industry Consortium" (PoC-CIC) was founded as an industry-driven organisation of device manufacturers, information system vendors and health care providers in early 2000 with the objective of connectivity between PoC analytical device devices and laboratory information systems (LIS). The resulting standard draft was transferred to the US NCCLS [4] standard body for publication as POCT1-A standard. It is expected to be adopted by CEN, ISO and IEEE in parallel.

For computerised electrocardiography, the ECG Standard Communications Protocol CEN ENV 1064 [5] specifies the exchange of data between ECG devices/carts and related computer systems. It provides a flexible data exchange format, a comprehensive coding scheme, and features like data compression etc. Due to the relevance of ECG data in numerous medical procedures and domains, however, diverse communication standards had to encompass ECG communication capabilities:

In the early eighties, IEEE (Institute of Electrical and Electronics Engineers) P1073 committee started work on standards for communication "primarily between bedside medical devices and patient care information systems, optimised for the acute care setting". Since 1993 a complementary set of European standards for point-of-care device communication was under development. CEN standards ENV 13734/35 [6] – commonly known under the acronym "VITAL" – and IEEE 1073 [7] documents have been aligned and supplemented to build the current CEN ISO/IEEE 11073 family of standards [8] to be further described in section 2.3.

1.2. Organisations in International e-Health Standardisation

For reasons mentioned above, established – nevertheless incompatible – healthcare communication standards were and are developed mostly independent of each other. Standardisation is performed by either national/international formal standard bodies or organisations of manufacturers and/or users [Figure 2]. Formal national standard bodies like AFNOR, ANSI, BSI, DIN, etc. are also responsible for the distribution of finalised standard documents within each country. The European Standardisation Organisation CEN is an umbrella organisation with regulative responsibility for standardisation within Europe. All EU countries participate by formal vote in the process of standard development. The relevant technical committee is TC 251 "Health Informatics" with its Working Group IV explicitly dedicated to "Technology for Interoperability". In ISO, the world-wide standard body, TC 215 deals with informatics issues in healthcare, Working Group 2 with "Messages and Communication". Various scientific organisations and manufacturer organisations have a strong interest in standardisation. They formed related groups either feeding their results into formal standardisation, like POCCIC did to NCCLS, or to publish them on their own, partly building organisation-specific systems of standards like DICOM. In the US, ANSI standardisation is generally based on various standard-developing organisations, each of them being responsible for a specific domain. Examples are lab-dedicated ASTM, HL7 and IEEE.

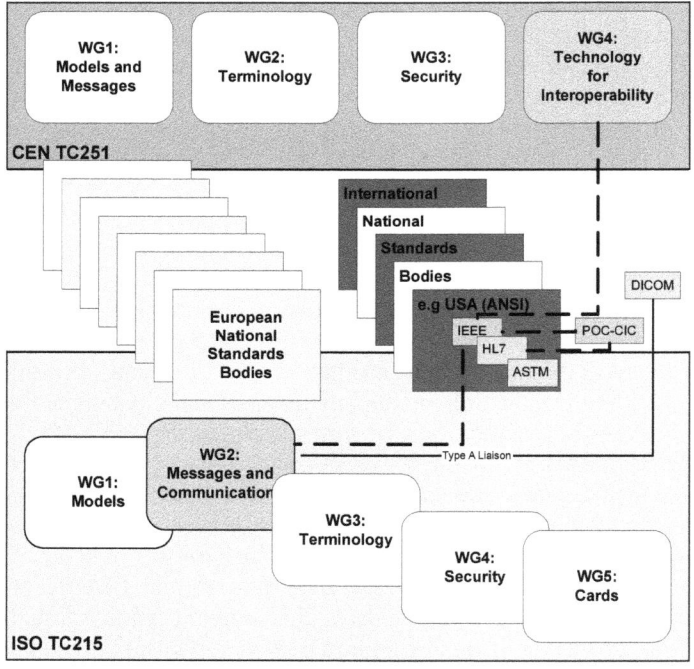

Figure 2. International "Health Informatics" standardisation organisations

1.3. Interoperability Concepts for Medical Devices

In contrast to other clinical communication standards, the CEN ISO/IEEE 11073 family of standards provides real-time "plug-and-play" interoperability to facilitate the efficient adding and swapping of acute and continuing care devices, such as patient monitors, ventilators, infusion pumps, ECG devices, etc in critical environment settings. To fulfil real-time requirements, a highly efficient "Medical Device Encoding" scheme is used. Conversion to alternative XML encoding reduces real-time capabilities, but enables use of XML-specific concepts and tools [9] promising dramatic cuts of development time and effort for interoperability component implementation. "Plug-

and-play" practically means that all the clinician has to do is make the connection – the systems automatically detect, configure and communicate without any subsequent human interaction, maintaining both functional and semantic interoperability.

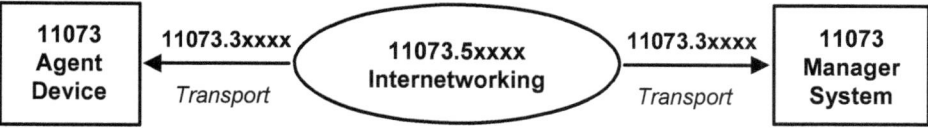

Figure 3. CEN ISO/IEEE 11073.5 Internetworking

Health informatics and clinical communication standards are often generally interpreted as relating to ISO/OSI Level 7 (HL7!) – based on the assumption of generally available LAN-infrastructure to build upon. For medical devices, interoperability explicitly implies all ISO/OSI Levels. While 11073 defines/modifies standards in ISO/OSI levels 7 – 5, it chiefly references to other standards (such as 802.x, IrDA, Bluetooth, etc.) in levels 1 – 4. For systems in homecare, even more for mobile systems which provide personal health services in dynamic environments, equivalent considerations apply. In order to enable functional interoperability using different (wired-, IR and RF wireless) network technologies, CEN ISO/IEEE 11073 provides standards for internetworking in the 11073.5 branch of the 11073 standards family. Figure 3 shows an 11073 "Agent Device", e.g. an infusion pump, pulse oximeter, or ventilator, and the corresponding 11073 "Manager System" – a patient monitor or device manager. Both are situated in different sub-networks using different network technologies. Other typical applications are wired-to-wireless transport gateways or LAN/IR access points.

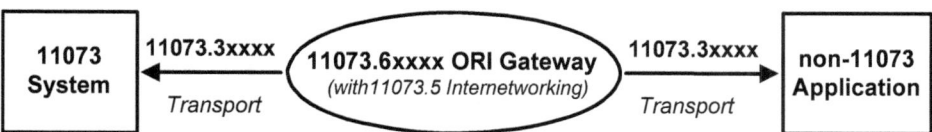

Figure 4. CEN ISO/IEEE 11075.6 Application Gateway

Based on CEN preparatory work [10], CEN ISO-IEEE 11073-60101 defines an 11073/HL7 "Observation Reporting interface" (ORI) enabling device-to-HIS-level interoperability (Figure 4). It is the first standard in the 11073.6 "Application Gateway" branch of the 11073 standards family which is intended to provide interoperability among different application protocols. The 11073 coding scheme is a registered HL7 Coding Scheme since 2003, permitting its use in HL7 messages.

1.4. Interoperability in the "Healthcare Enterprise"

Apart from formal standardisation activities increasingly addressing cross-standard interoperability issues, the IHE ("Integrating the Healthcare Enterprise") initiative [11] initiated in 1998 by HIMSS (Healthcare Information and Management Systems Society) and RSNA (Radiological Society of North America) embarks on a complementary strategy to "promote and support the integration of systems in a healthcare enterprise (hospital)". Motivated by the obvious lack of interoperability among available HIS, RIS or PACS systems, clinical workflow optimisation (e.g. to provide continuity and integrity of patient information, to foster communication among information systems from different vendors, to avoid repeating tasks like typing patient names, to eliminate data redundancy etc.) is maintained by a set of "Integration Profiles" which specify the use of existing standards. Part of the IHE work on DICOM/HL7 interoperability is equivalent to the CEN ISO/IEEE 11073-60101 ORI standard. Ongoing IHE work aims at integrating Laboratory/Point-of-Care Testing and ECG communication.

2. Ubiquitous Personal Health Services – "pHealth"

2.1. Personal Health Service Access Paradigm

During the last century, the ways individuals could access health services did not change significantly until the last decade: Patients had to personally contact their GP or other health professional for advice or treatment, or to indicate an emergency by phone. Hospital resources (specialised expertise, intervention and care services) defining the second/top level of health services could only be accessed by admission. Health professionals in different institutions used to communicate by paper letters. With electronic data processing and data communications becoming available, trans-institutional applications like teleconsultation, teleconferencing and remote decision support were introduced, but their use was limited to clinical environments.

The development of microprocessors resulted in widespread use of personal computers among all institutions involved in professional healthcare. In the personal health area, it enabled applications like remotely monitored homecare. The "telematics" concept, generally indicating the fusion of telecommunication and information processing technologies, was adopted and extended to "health telematics". Ongoing "health telematics infrastructure" implementation is regarded to enable eHealth. From a patient perspective, personal EHR-based applications could not only provide information and feedback fostering patient compliance, but also make privately acquired information available to health professionals. For the time being, access to health-related information and services is mainly provided by Internet access. Quality and interpretation of Internet-derived information, however, depend on the user's competence and skills.

Future ubiquitous personal health scenarios clearly reach beyond the paradigms and concepts of "eHealth" (Figure 5). They imply continuous location-independent access to personalised health-related information, assistance, support and intervention, enabling applications like continuous monitoring of personal health status, or health-status-related stepwise activation of hierarchically cooperating services and functions (rings in Figure 5). Implementing such an escalation strategy can help avoiding inefficient and inadequate use of resources. In case of emergency, the remote service receiving the alarm can switch BAN operation mode to real-time-transmission of BAN-delivered vital signs waveform data (e.g. ECG) and in parallel derive relevant demographic and patient history information from distributed EHR repositories. Thus ambulance and hospital staff can be optimally prepared for further patient treatment.

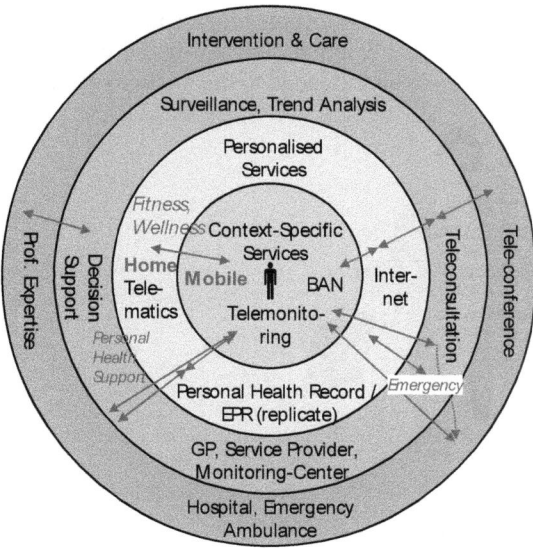

Figure 5. Multi-Level Personal Health Service Access Scheme

2.2. The Body Area Network Concept

The Body Area Network (BAN) concept specifies wireless communication between several miniaturised, intelligent Body Sensor (or actuator) Units (BSU) and a single Body Central Unit (BCU) worn at the human body. It is characterised by a maximum range typical for human body dimensions, e.g. 2m.

The BCU concentrates the BSU-originating data streams, performs intermediate storage and processing as well as communication to the outside world using standard wireless technology like DECT, WLAN or Bluetooth. The Network Access Unit (NAU) can be implemented as a medical gateway hosting an embedded web-server.

Both NAU and BCU may provide standard interfaces, particularly implementing 11073 "Agent" functionality. From a communication perspective, a BAN can thus be regarded equivalent to a 11073-compliant modular medical device, implying semantic interoperability between BAN and remote professional or clinical systems.

2.3. IMEX – a Micro-System Perspective for Interoperability

As development of micro-sensors and micro-systems particularly for homecare and personal health-related applications is progressing, acquisition of multiple biosignals, for instance blood pressure (BP), ECGs, respiration, urine flow etc. can be performed by means of miniaturised patient-worn equipment. Utilising the BAN concept for collection and communication of data to enable multi-parameter monitoring, micro-sensors can also be integrated into BSU units.

The German IMEX project [12] aimed at communication among micro-systems and with external device systems analysing possible interfaces and their communication requirements. Accordingly a Micro System Data format (MSD) was defined which enables the use of standard health telematics coding schemes for semantic core elements on micro-system-level, minimising processing overhead for preparation of micro-system-generated data for external standard-based communication. Thus the "semantic interoperability chain" is extended to the micro-system level.

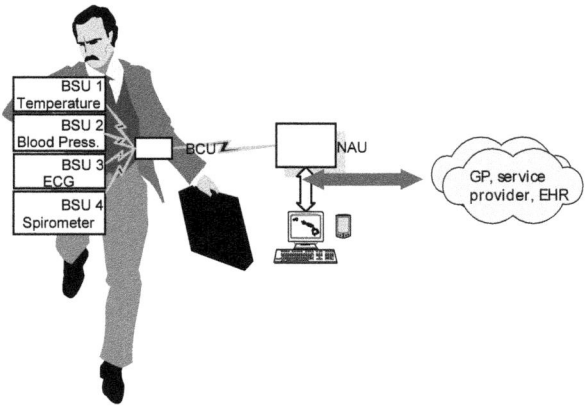

Figure 6. BAN concept and components

3. Conclusions

"Interoperability" implies a number of different concepts, e.g. Functional Interoperability and Internetworking, Semantic Interoperability and Application Gateways. Health information integration ("eHealth") established a demand for interoperability between clinical and healthcare-related stakeholders, systems and processes or workflows. Domain-specific communication and interoperability standards are well established, but have to be supplemented for trans-domain use. Interoperability concepts for medical devices as well as for personal and/or mobile systems need to involve all 7 ISO/OSI reference model layers and particularly have to include terminology/coding aspects.

The advanced concept of "pHealth" extends "eHealth" by the inclusion of smart sensors, body-worn mobile systems and situation-specific activation of applications and human health professionals, thus providing personalised ubiquitous health services. Body Area Networks and micro-systems are building blocks of future personalised health telematics infrastructures that extend existing interoperability concepts.

References

[1]   IEEE Standard Computer Dictionary - A Compilation of IEEE Standard Computer Glossaries, 1990
[2]   http://www.hl7.org
[3]   http://medical.nema.org/
[4]   http://www.nccls.org or http://www.clsi.org
[5]   http://www.centc251.org
[6]   http://www.ieee1073.org
[7]   http://www.iso.ch/tc215
[8]   http://www.w3.org/

[9]　CEN SSS-HIDE (2001): Health Informatics-Strategies for harmonisation and integration of device-level and enterprise-wide methodologies for communication as applied to HL7, LOINC and ENV 13734, see [6]

[10]　http://www.rsna.org/ihe

[11]　Becks T, Dehm J.: IMEX – A New Knowledge Platform for Microsystems in Medicine. http://www.vde-mikromedizin.de

[12]　http://www.iec.ch/

IV. Community Health 1

Personalised Health Management Systems
C.D. Nugent et al. (Eds.)
IOS Press, 2005

Homecare Service Perspective in Tuscany: Vision and New User Centred Services

Cristiano PAGGETTI and Elena TAMBURINI

MEDEA – Medical Engineering and Applications, Florence, Italy

Abstract. "With medical knowledge expanding every day, no physician can keep up without help. By using high-tech medical communication, high-performance computers, high resolution video, and fibre-optic information "superhighways," we have been able to put the entire world of medical science at the fingertips of even the most isolated rural family doctor." [1] This quote by a former Surgeon General encapsulates the promise and potential for healthcare technology. Service organization and stakeholders' commitment are the real crucial issues for actual e-Health services deployment. In such a contest Homecare services start playing such a role of services integration and new care models development.

Keywords. Homecare, Personalized Healthcare, Smart Home, Care Models.

Introduction

Several steps must be undertaken to speed up e-Health service deployment. Table 1 [1] summarizes the issues which are considered related to the improvement of healthcare quality. The strategies illustrated in Table 1 have to comply with cost reduction of overall healthcare and social expenditures, combined optimization and integration of services. Table 2 [3] summarizes issues related to reduction of healthcare costs. As can be seen from Tables 1 and 2 the scenario shows a high level of complexity and a multitude of factors affecting the overall result. Nowadays healthcare can benefit from telecommunication technology as well as from integration of technologies such as assistive technology, wearable sensors, miniaturized remote sensing and delivering devices focused not only on treatment but on prevention, education, self care and improvement of independent living. Service organization and stakeholders' commitment are the real crucial issues for actual e-Health services deployment. Indeed services and remote assistance provided by Homecare platforms are perceived by people and stakeholders as relevant approaches to improve healthcare quality. In particular if we refer to cost reduction analysis it is relevant to take into account the research conducted by the Università Cattolica in Rome. This research showed that Homecare services could represent an efficient and strategic approach combined with cost saving figures. In fact, it was reported that hospitalization costs an average of 500 euro per day per person whereas Homecare services cost an average of 50 euro per day per person. The research identified market related drivers such as:

- Increasing demand for homeland security and public health technologies.
- Rapidly increasing demand for Homecare.
- Increasing acceptance by medical professionals and institutions of e-Health services.

Nevertheless, the research study indicated that hospitalization is still the most frequent solution applied.

1. Personalized Homecare Prospective

In the personalized healthcare domain it is necessary to mature a specific vision for the definition and expedition of a new paradigm of integrated social healthcare services able to address three fundamental goals:

1.   The improvement of people's health and wellbeing,
2.   People's satisfaction and participation in their own healthcare,
3.   Services efficiency and sustainability.

Table 1. Method and strategies to improve healthcare quality.

GOALS	METHODS	INVESTMENTS	POSSIBLES INCENTIVES
Reduce illness	Disease management	Payer incentives for disease management	Bonus payments or investment credits to providers for applying quality improvement technologies
		Preventive medicine programs	Individual tax credits or subsidies for enrolling patients in preventive maintenance programs
		Information technology	Accelerated depreciation on disease management devices and applications
	Professional and patient education	e-Learning infrastructure and applications	Individual or business tax credits for program enrolment/development
Reduce hospitalization	Homecare	Adoption of: Devices and applications Information technology	Accelerated depreciation on Homecare devices and applications; Expanded Medicare/Medicaid reimbursement for monitoring services
	Remote monitoring	Adoption of: Devices and applications Information technology	Accelerated depreciation on remote monitoring devices and applications; Expanded Medicare/Medicaid reimbursement for monitoring services; Bonus payments or tax credits for reduced hospitalization rates and reduced outpatient visits

Table 2. Method and strategies to reduce of healthcare costs.

GOALS	METHODS	INVESTMENTS	PERFORMANCE MEASURES and POSSIBLES INCENTIVES
Automate administration	Adopt information technology	Rationalization of Reimbursement policies;	Awards, recognition and other incentives for effective cost reduction programs;
		Automation of administrative operations	Expanded investment tax credits or accelerated depreciation for automation expenses;
			Low-interest loans for automation
Integrate applications	Software interoperability and systems integration	Systems integration	Metrics related to cost reduction such as change in costs per encounter;
			Tax policy which incentives cost reduction and use of metrics
	Education and training	Professional training programs	Certification programs for healthcare technology integrators/professionals
Increase productivity	Adopt information technology	Financial data systems and applications; Develop and adopt applications for measuring productivity	Metrics related to productivity such as number of total staff hours per encounter or total costs per encounter; Design and implement tax policies which incentives productivity measurement
	Education and training	Needs assessment Curricula development e-Learning programs	Formal recognition for productivity gains resulting from e-Health investments
Share resources	Technology cooperatives	Awareness campaign to include "best practices;" Establish buyer "co-ops;" Practice demand aggregation	Favourable tax treatment for buyer cooperatives or for sharing technology resources
Increase return on investment		Create business and return on investment models; Undertake data collection/surveys; Undertake cost-benefit analyses	Industry indices/benchmarks

These goals could be addressed in several scenarios by means of different platforms. In such a context Homecare, defined as the provision of services at home based on assistive technologies integrated in a stable communication infrastructure and delivered through an integrated network of stakeholders, provides the concrete framework for realization of these three aims.

Homecare not only represents a model of integrated, permanent and personalized service, based on a user centred approach, it in addition implements a multi agent, multi services, multiple devices, multi channel and knowledge based solution.

Wearable sensors, remote-monitoring devices and knowledge management agents are only a part of the overall levels interacting in such a domain.

In Figure 1 [4] the home evolution concept is represented which combines new home products and solutions with services, including Homecare, all supported vai a global area network basis.

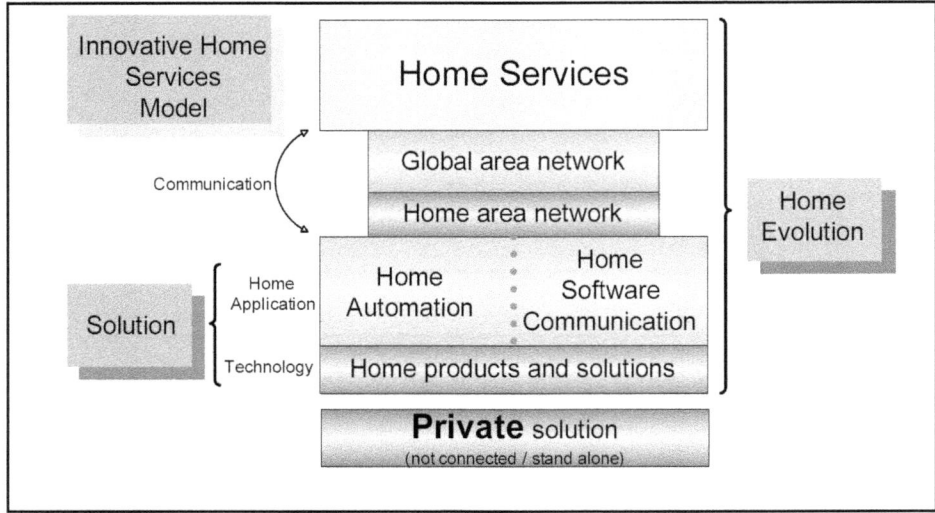

Figure 1. Home Evolution Components.

Taking into account e-Health and personalized Health domains, several projects and pilots have identified specific users' and stakeholders' needs, ICT components and have expedited market acceptance for several e-Health solutions. Nevertheless, the most crucial issue is the fact there is a severe lack of well-established care models and stakeholders' collaboration schemes to exploit e-Health solutions.

User needs analysis shows that there is a severe gap between emerging technology solutions and users' expectations and basic needs. In particular innovation is declared as a factor of secondary importance, yet the stakeholders require an improvement in terms of security, standardization and interoperable solutions.

Table 3 presents the issues of Primary and Secondary importance to a range of stakeholders in relation to e-Health solutions.

In such a framework Homecare stands out as an approach able to promote an integration of hospital healthcare and assistance at home. Homecare improves homeland security, access to services, enables diagnosis and clinical advice based on specialists operating remotely and improves then timeliness of care by providing a means of social and clinical data sharing among stakeholder groups. In addition, Homecare reduces the commuting between home and hospital.

Table 3. The issues of Primary and Secondary importance to stakeholders.

STAKEHOLDERS	Homeland Security	Access	Quality	Cost	Innovation	Competitiveness
Homeland Security	P[1]	P	P	P	P	S[2]
First Responders	P	P	P	P	S	S
Public Health	P	P	P	P	S	S
Military	P	P	P	P	P	S
Clinicians	S	S	P	P	S	P
Payers	S	S	P	P	S	P
Consumer	P	P	P	P	S	S
e-Health Manufacturers/Vendors	S	S	P	P	P	P

However, it is implicit in the Homecare approach that it is necessary to define a new organizational and collaborative care model among different stakeholders. In fact it is not the technology per se which is the key success but it is how the service satisfies user's needs, how the user's training is conducted and how the service is integrated in the local Social/Healthcare service provision protocol. As a consequence two main features must be fulfilled by Homecare platforms:

- A dynamic level of involvement of the different stakeholders and users within the care model.
- A flexible service architecture that can be applied in different scenarios according to different healthcare models and regulatory frameworks.

2. Homecare Service Perspective in Tuscany and Italy

There is an emerging requirement to improve the quality of life at home in terms of personal autonomy, inclusion in society, communication facilities, entertainment, self-care, safety and cost savings in home management.

In Italy there is a growing development and testing of new Homecare services. Such experiences are related to the National Healthcare Programme (PSN 2003-2005) that promotes Homecare as a root for the implementation of appropriate and efficient care pathways for prevention and continuity of care.

The Tuscany Region addresses the ambitious goal of guaranteeing social and healthcare services by a means of participation of public and private institutions and citizens in the services organization and management.

In Tuscany a concrete strategy has been put in place to converge several international experiences and resources in multidisciplinary approaches (cultural, social, technological and methodological domains) for Homecare services development. The strategy is focused on involvement of public institutions, citizens and healthcare operators, enterprises, voluntary associations and research centres.

---

[1] P = Primary
[2] S = Secondary

In such a scenario, acting as solutions providers and system integrators in several e-Health services, we have developed our vision of Homecare service provision that can be summarised as follows:

- The customer as a person

- The product as a service

- The service "designed and tested" by the person

The approach we have developed combines modular basis healthcare assistance, social support and independent living, providing the user with an integrated portfolio of services.

As a result we have implemented a specific service model development methodology for the definition and start-up of Homecare services in Tuscany.

The proposed approach as summarised in Table 4 combines in a single coherent vision cultural, sociological, technological and methodological domains.

Table 4. Service model development approach.

Component	Question addressed
Patient Population Specific to the site	What are the characteristics and needs of the patient group?
Essential service elements necessary to deliver e-Health at that site	What clinical resources are necessary to support these patients at home?
Technology Requirements recommended	What technology is necessary to support the clinical needs?
Weave above steps together into a service design concept	How do the essential service elements and technology fit together?

In the following sections two real examples of Homecare Services in Tuscany are presented. Such examples and other e-Health experiences of cooperation among different stakeholders insist in the overall infrastructural telematics project of the Tuscany region. On such a network infrastructure both private and public institutions can operate as users as well as services providers.

2.1. Telecare Platform

The Telecare platform involves 2,500 users and sets up an ***innovative Home Care service model,*** exploiting potential and synergies of different technologies (home automation, wearable devices, assistive technologies and telemedicine).

The user's home is equipped with a Set Top Box unit acting as a home HUB for different data and requests (Figure 2). The Set Top Box enables the TV to become the user's interface for a set of bidirectional services to be selected by the TV remote controller.

By this means the unique user interface provided by the Set Top Box allows the user to operate assistive technologies, engage with home automation solutions, control remote vital signal monitoring devices and access entertainment,   social and educational services. In addition the users can establish a videoconference with family members, other users or Service Centre operators.

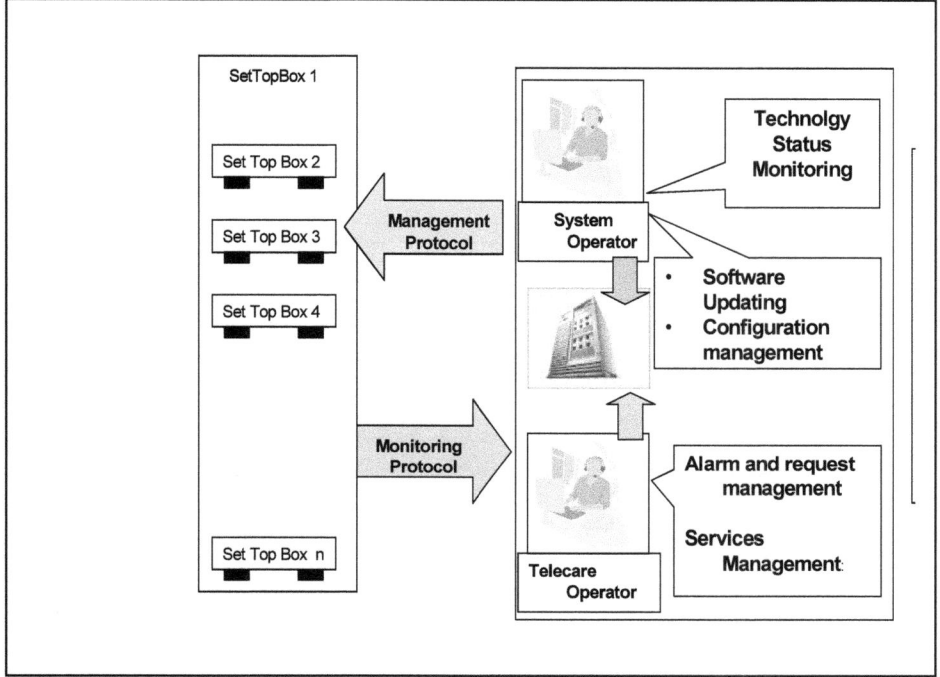

Figure 2. Telecare Platform: Functional components Architecture.

The Telecare Service Centre is equipped with the web platform DG-HOME that enables operators to perform real time monitoring and management of each user's requests, their agenda, their environment and personal alarms in a *cooperative environment* and can all be shared by different stakeholders and caregivers.

The DG-HOME functionalities are based on a remote solving problem approach and *personalized home care solution management,* through the remote monitoring of each user's requests and the real time availability of user's data (clinical records and contact information). Figure 3 shows a typical example of screen information from the application.

According to a structured and personalized *data management approach,* specific protocols allow the management of the following services through a multi-channel communication platform (telephone, instant messaging, video-conference):

- Remote management of user's alarms (security and safety requirements).
- Tele-monitoring of clinical parameters (i.e. ECG signal, blood pressure, drugs compliance).
- Tele-support and remote management of the user's agenda.
- e-Government services.
- Communication with social and health Service Centre (i.e. pharmacies, GPs, hospitals, public administrations).
- Alarm and Request Management according with personalized protocol.

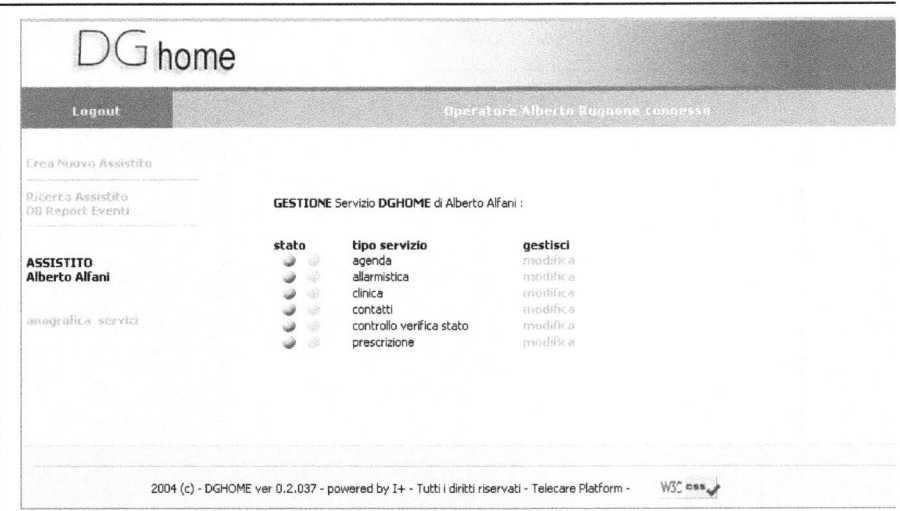

Figure 3. DGHome Platform: Alarm and Request Management according to personalized protocol.

2.2. DOMUS – Personalized Home Evolution and Service Design

DOMUS is a project funded by the Tuscany Region. A domestic environment has been equipped with assistive devices, home automation solutions and networking services available on the market.

The goal of the DOMUS service is to let the user, mainly people with physical disabilities, test different Homecare solutions and through specific training let them identify solutions able to improve their independent living (Figure 4).

After two weeks of training an interdisciplinary team designs and verifies with the user a personalized Homecare solution and services portfolio. The ensuing step is to install and activate such services at the patient's own home.

During the training and at the patient's home the Service Centre, through the DG-Home platform, provides the remote management of requests and alarms, involving also healthcare operators, providers of social and emergency services and local voluntary associations.

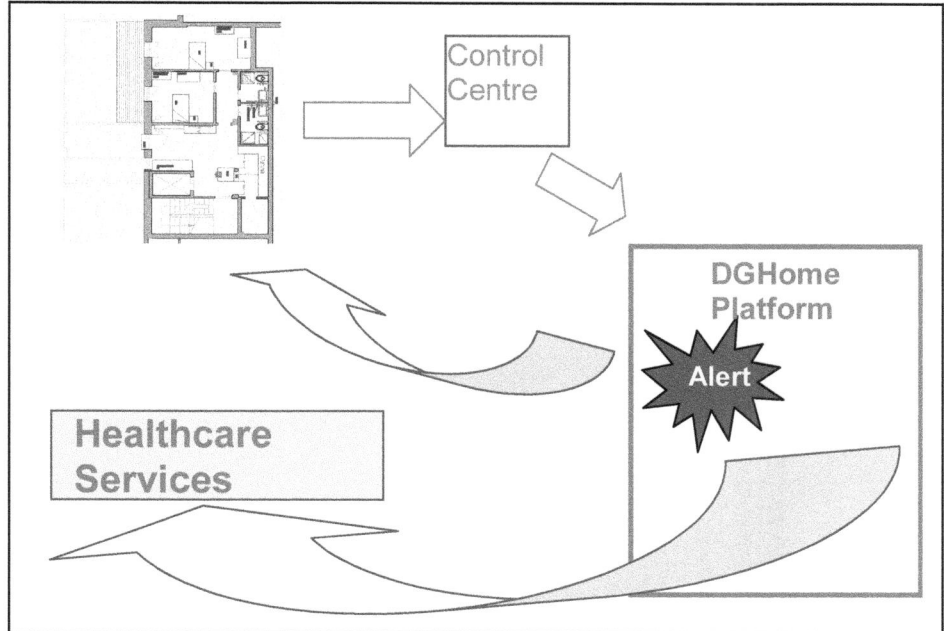

Figure 4. Domus Architectural components.

3. Conclusion

Today we are dealing with quite mature e-Health solutions and evolving technologies with the real challenge being to develop, manage and assess new care models.

The European Commission itself, in the past ten years has funded several projects and initiatives aimed to develop new e-Health solutions, and nowadays is promoting the adoption of Homecare services and is funding best practice dissemination and e-Health service assessment.

e-Health best practice results and assessment reports are presented to key players and a coordination among planners, policy-makers, researchers and program managers is promoted to insure the most efficient, integrated strategies for increasing e-Health services access, improving quality and reducing costs, and for assuring that public policy reflects current services issues and opportunities, is adopted.

Pursuing a similar approach Homecare could play a central role in the social and healthcare framework. Homecare is able to promote innovative care models and e-inclusion approaches exploiting networking infrastructures providing an integrated portfolio of high quality services based on cost effectiveness and a sustainable basis.

References

[1] Koop Institute web site http://www.dartmouth.edu/dms/koop/projects/past/nnehii.shtml C. Everett Koop, M.D.

[2]   "Innovation, Demand and Investment in Telehealth" U.S. Department of Commerce Office of Technology Policy February 2004.
[3]   "Innovation, Demand and Investment in Telehealth" U.S. Department of Commerce Office of Technology Policy February 2004.
[4]   "Da domotica a Home Evolution: tecnologie, sistemi e servizi integrati per la casa e l'abitare" Roberto Taranto ANIE Milano 11/9/04.

Personalised Health Management Systems
C.D. Nugent et al. (Eds.)
IOS Press, 2005

A Cataract Decision Support System: its Requirement is Increasing

Johnny MOORE

Department of Ophthalmology, Royal Victoria Hospital , Northern Ireland

Abstract. Cataract surgery and intraocular lens implantation has taken on many significant advances since its earliest inception. As the prevalence of the aged population increases the number of cataract operations also increases year on year. In the UK last year over 300,000 cataract operations were performed with 2 million in Europe and 1.5 million in the USA. Globally 8.7 million cataract operations are performed per annum. Technical advances are occurring ever more rapidly in this procedure enabling improved preoperative assessment and surgical management. This has produced a sophisticated procedure which is eminently reproducible. In concordance with such improvements both patient and doctors expectations for visual results have also risen. The expectation is now that the operation will achieve more than mere removal of a pathological opacity interfering with the visual process. The possibility and expectation is that the procedure will be tailored specifically to the patient in such a way that the best possible visual result will be achieved through customization of the surgical process to optimize the individual's optical system. Optimization of any particular process may be complex, and cataract surgery is no exception. Careful consideration of many interrelated factors including a patient's functional visual requirements, along with specific anatomical and unique optical factors will be required if an optimum result is to be achieved. The decision making process involved in determining how an individual eye should be surgically customised, can therefore be complicated. These are the situations where decision support systems become most beneficial, to ensure consistent successful results, particularly if technical measurements are being performed by individuals with varying degrees of experience.

Keywords. Cataract Surgery, Decision Support.

Introduction

The word cataract originates from the Greek word for waterfall. In early times it was thought that a cataract flowed like a waterfall within the eye with white water blindness representing cataract and black water blindness representing glaucoma. The earliest reference within the literature to a cataract is found in Sanskrit manuscripts dating to 5th century BC. The type of operation practiced then was couching where the lens was forcibly pushed back into the vitreous. This resulted in improved vision initially but subsequent visual loss due to chronic ocular inflammation or retinal detachments.

In the western world the first written description of a cataract extraction was in 29AD in De Medicinae the work of Latin encyclopaedist Celsus. Modern cataract surgery where the cataract is removed from the eye was introduced by Jacques Daviel in Paris in 1748. This was further adapted by the introduction of sutures to the operation in 1867 by Willard Willimas in Boston. It was in the 1940s before Harold Ridley introduced the intraocular lens. Another major advance in intracapsular surgery was in 1957 when Barraquer from Spain introduced alpha-chymotrypsin to dissolve the zonules for lens removal, the chemical though successfully used for many years is no longer commercially available. Krawicz of Poland in 1961 introduced the use of a cryosurgical probe to facilitate intracapsular lens extraction by freezing attachment of the cryoprobe to the superior cataract surface. The 1960s have heralded the most significant recent alteration in cataract surgery technique through the introduction by Charles Kelman of ultrasound designed to emulsify cataracts and allow their removal through very small diameter incisions. This has facilitated more rapid rehabilitation of the eye post surgical intervention and is now the main technique practiced in modern ophthalmic centres throughout the world.

1. The Human Crystalline Lens

The primary function of the human crystalline lens is to refract light passing through the cornea to focus onto the retina. The young crystalline lens also allows alteration of its shape to change the vergence ability and hence enable accommodation to view both distant and near objects on demand. The human lens changes constantly throughout life. It is shaped like an oblate spheroid, with anterior and posterior surfaces whose shape can be described as paraboloid with a steeper curvature located centrally near the optical axis and with surfaces which become progressively flatter towards the mid periphery. The lens increases in mass and size throughout life, however MRI measurements show no change in the accommodated lens diameters with age [1]. In vivo Scheimpflug measurements of unaccommodated eyes indicate that the anterior and posterior lens surfaces increase in curvature with increasing age [2]. The resultant optical effect from this change of shape is an age dependant increase in spherical aberration induced by the lens. In fact on average in the population the lens has negative spherical aberration at age 10 which becomes zero by age 40 and positive thereafter [3]. These changes are important with regard to visual function and partly explain the decrease in visual function with age. Irrespective of cataract, vision deteriorates with the aging population. Corneal shape changes little with age while the lens alters its shape as outlined above. In young people there appears to be a balance between positive spherical aberrations induced by the cornea and negative spherical aberrations produced by the lens, which results in improved visual acuity; this affect however is increasingly lost with age [4].

Spectacles have been used for at least 700 years to correct both defocus and astigmatism. Many other visual aberrations, however, are present in the eye in addition to these two aberrations. Until recently it has not been possible to either measure or treat aberrations other than the traditional defocus and astigmatism. Recent advances in refractive surgery have led to instruments both capable of accurately measuring higher order aberrations both from the corneal surface and total eye wavefront aberrations. These are being increasingly utilized within clinical practice to measure ocular higher order aberrations which if large can be treated through laser refractive techniques. Prior to refractive surgery little attention was given to wavefront aberration mainly because in normal eyes, even with large pupils, vision is usually not degraded significantly below 6/6 vision. With the advent of refractive surgery, however, often very large amounts of spherical aberration and coma were induced secondary to the refractive procedure.

2. Clinical Assessment Procedures

The clinical tools now used to measure ocular wavefront aberration, are based upon either the technique of interferometry or ray tracing. Interferometers work by firstly splitting light and recombining it after its divided beams have been reflected by both reference and target surface. Only if the surfaces are identical and correctly aligned will no interference fringes be visible, otherwise the resulting fringe pattern provides a topographic map of the wave aberration. Interferometry is, however, a little used method due to associated technical difficulties. Most clinical instruments used therefore are based upon the principal of ray tracing and reconstruction of the wave aberration by integrating the slopes of the individual rays of light imaged in the pupillary plane. The aberration map which is formed at the level of the pupil is similar in concept to corneal topographic maps designed to describe the corneal shape. The difference between them is that the cornea map describes curvature while the aberration map describes the difference between a wavefront of light and a reference wavefront. The use of mathematical formula to create aberration maps and to display them in easily identifiable ways has been greatly facilitated through the use of two distinct mathematical techniques. These are Fourier analysis and Zernike analysis, Zernike having more recently replaced Fourier as the principal method to describe aberrations within the field of refractive and cataract surgery [5]. These polynomials are used to define aberrations in a form which can be programmed into a laser computer to allow their treatment and removal from the optical pathway within a specific eye by changing the surface of the cornea to counteract the total aberration.

Zernike equations can be derived using Hamilton's equations and are depicted in Eq. (1).

$$\phi^{(4)} = -\frac{1}{4}A\rho^4 - Bx_0^2\rho^2\cos^2\theta - \frac{1}{2}Cx_0^2\rho^2 + Dx_0\rho\cos\theta + Ex_0\rho^3\cos\theta \qquad (1)$$

where ρ is the distance of the object ray from the z-axis, and the fourth order of the aberration wavefront is where it appears to be applicable to human vision. At present it is thought that any higher would essentially be inconsequential. Future research may, however, prove that higher order aberrations are also clinically important.

Each of the coefficients in the wavefront represents a different defect in the eye:

A = Spherical Aberration
B = Coma
C = Astigmatism
D = Curvature of Field
E = Distortion

The wavefront aberration can be separated into X3 and Y3 components:

$$X_3 = A\rho^3 \cos\theta + Bx_0\rho^2(2 + \cos 2\theta) + (3C + D)x_0^2\rho\cos\theta + Ex_0^3$$
$$Y_3 = A\rho^3 \sin\theta + Bx_0\rho^2 \sin 2\theta + (C + D)x_0^2\rho\sin\theta$$

which are the aberration components of lowest order. The axes are chosen so the x, z-plane passes through the object point thus y0 = 0.

The first three of these aberrations are present in everyone's eye to some degree but it is only when any of the coefficients become particularly large that they cause evident problems. Generally, due to aging of the eye, these coefficients will automatically increase but often it is not enough to have a profound effect on vision.

Using the above equations if all the coefficients, except A, are zeroed what remains represents spherical aberration. The equation representing spherical aberration is outlined below:

$$X_3 = A\rho^3 \cos\theta$$
$$Y_3 = A\rho^3 \sin\theta$$

Looking at this one can recognise that;

$$(X_3^2 + Y_3^2) = (A\rho^3)^2$$

This is clearly the equation of a circle with centre (0,0) and radius Aρ3, which tells us that object rays that strike the eye at a constant distance ρ intersect the image plane in a circle of radius Aρ3, so the image of a point is seen as a circle on the retina. It follows that close to the centre of the image focus is sharp as the value of ρ would be very small. The edges of the image would be blurred because each point would be seen as quite a large circle as the value of ρ increases. Waves passing near the centre of the cornea and lens are refracted slightly but those at the periphery are refracted to a greater degree creating hazy edges, thus the blur is relative to the centre of the object.

The peripheral and axial rays are not in common focus but the circle of least confusion is defined as the place where the rays come closest to focusing together i.e. the area of the smallest diameter.

2.1. Coma

If all the coefficients are set equal to zero except B the resulting aberration is known as coma. This is the first off axis aberration. The X3 and Y3 values are defined as:

$$X_3 = Bx_0\rho^2(2+\cos 2\theta)$$
$$Y_3 = Bx_0\rho^2 \sin 2\theta$$

Combining these we get:

$$(X_3 - 2Bx_0\rho^2)^2 + Y_3^2 = (Bx_0\rho^2)^2$$

This again is the equation of a circle centre ($2Bx_0\rho^2$,0) and radius $Bx_0\rho^2$. So similarly to spherical aberration each point is seen as a circle of radius $Bx_0\rho^2$ so the smaller the value of ρ the clearer the image. The circles have a common tangent; the angle subtended by the two tangents at the x-axis is 30° so the image is confined between two lines subtending angles of 30° in the x-direction.

Since the centre of the circle is ($2Bx_0\rho^2$,0) the point spread function is even greater than that of spherical aberration as it is off the axis.

So as ρ increases the image radius increases and the centre of the image shifts away from the paraxial image point giving an almost triangular spread. Blur is directed away from the optic axis. The image created has a 'comet-like' appearance hence why the aberration is called coma.

It is coma and spherical aberration that are the most crippling visual defects because singular points spread so much that they end up overlapping each other creating unrecognisable hazy images.

2.2. The Intraocular Lens

How each type of aberration will functionally effect an individual patient, however, is related as much to their functional visual requirements as to the exact optics of their eye.

A plethora of lens designs and materials have now entered the field of cataract and refractive surgery, far removed from the early days when Harold Ridley implanted the first intraocular lens in 1951 in St Thomas's hospital London. The advances in lenses have been principally led by manufacturing companies whose design changes have occurred in tandem to the demands of improved surgical technique. Small incision surgery developed through the work of Charles Kelman on phaocemulsification, has generated an increasing requirement for intraocular lenses able to pass through ever smaller incisions yet still retain optimal optical properties. Which is the optimal lens type or design for each individual patient is as yet, however, difficult to determine, with few clinical trials sufficiently robustly designed and implemented to differentiate between intraocular lens types, material or design.

At present the materials used include:-silicone, acrylic polymers designed to produce a hydrophobic or hydrophilic intraocular lens, HEMA, PMMA and other combinations and variations in material. Recently a subtle design change in intraocular lenses has occurred 'across the industry' in order to reduce posterior capsular opacification. The posterior edge profile of the intraocular lens has been changed from a round to a square edge and this has significantly reduced posterior capsular opacification rates, at least for the early postoperative period. Certain lens manufacturers have in addition targeted the anterior lens surface shape changing it to become more prolate shaped to reduce spherical aberration. Recent attempts to produce mechanically designed intraocular lenses that will mimic the natural lens physiology of allowing lenses to increase power on demand to allow focus for near vision have resulted in various designs. None of these, however, have been proven to be fully effective, with significant inter-individual variation in accommodative effect [6]. This variation makes it difficult to accurately predict what each individual patient will achieve. Significant improvements with regard to design and manufacture of intraocular lenses are still required before achievement of adequate sustainable accommodative function in all patients is reached. Multifocal intraocular lenses (MIOLs) provide a further option to provide distant and near vision without the use of spectacle aids [7]. Gimbal reported on 149 patients with a bilateral 3M diffractive MIOLs and found that 63% of these patients did not require spectacle correction for near vision compared to 4% with monofocal intraocular lenses. Multifocal patients however do report greater visual side-effects such as glare, haloes and loss of contrast sensitivity [8]. Again the ability to predict which patients will benefit most from one form of surgery or another or who will be most likely to suffer from unwanted visual side-effects requires significantly more research. Patient satisfaction with the MIOLs is more likely if surgeons and technical staff follow inclusion and exclusion criteria for patient selection and surgeons learn to reduce any unwanted astigmatism [9].

3. Conclusion

The importance of specific patient and operative data collection and analysis is becoming increasingly recognised within the field of customised refractive cataract surgery [10]. It is imperative, however, that a greater understanding is achieved as to which factors are important and are truly predictive of improved functional outcomes. This information will allow the development of treatment algorithms which will allow proper customisation of the treatment process for each patient. To help achieve this, the author in conjunction with the University of Ulster is creating a self-learning database integrated within the cataract clinical pathway from outpatient pre-assessment through surgery to postoperative review. This database combines objective and subjective patient data to provide relevant information required to advise on treatment algorithms designed to improve patient outcomes. A decision support system which integrates and uses this database is being designed for outpatient and theatre environments. The aim of this process is to assist and improve cataract training and to enable and confirm clinical results. The decision support system incorporates basic artificial intelligence linked through the web to all major search engines and relevant clinical databases to ensure that clinical advice given is correlated both with specific surgical results and with the constantly updated ophthalmic literature.

References

[1]   Strenk SA, Semmlow JL, Strenk LM, Munoz P, Gronlund-Jacob J, DeMarco JK. Age-related changes in human ciliary muscle and lens: a magnetic resonance imaging study.Invest Ophthalmol Vis Sci. 1999 May;40(6):1162-9.
[2]   Koretz JF, Handelman GH, Brown NP.Analysis of human crystalline lens curvature as a function of accommodative state and age.Vision Res. 1984;24(10):1141-51.

[3]   Glasser A, Campbell MC.Presbyopia and the optical changes in the human crystalline lens with age. Vision Res. 1998 Jan;38(2):209-29

[4]   Fujikado T, Kuroda T, Ninomiya S, Maeda N, Tano Y, Oshika T, Hirohara Y,Mihashi T.Age-related changes in ocular and corneal aberrations.Am J Ophthalmol. 2004 Jul;138(1):143-6.

[5]   Klyce SD, Karon MD, Smolek MK.Advantages and disadvantages of the Zernike expansion for representing wave aberration of the normal and aberrated eye. J Refract Surg. 2004 Sep-Oct;20(5):S537-41

[6]   Dick HB.Accommodative intraocular lenses: current status.Curr Opin Ophthalmol. 2005 Feb;16(1):8-26.

[7]   Bellucci R.Multifocal intraocular lenses., Curr Opin Ophthalmol. 2005 Feb;16(1):33-7.

[8]   Javitt JC, Steinert RF. Cataract extraction with multifocal intraocular lens implantation: a multinational clinical trial evaluating clinical, functional, and quality-of-life outcomes,Ophthalmology. 2000 Nov;107(11):2040-8..

[9]   Steinert RF. Visual outcomes with multifocal intraocular lenses.Curr Opin Ophthalmol. 2000 Feb;11(1):12-21.

[10] Aslam TM, Gilmour D, Hopkinson S, Patton N, Aspinall P. The development and assessment of a self-perceived quality of vision questionnaire to test pseudophakic patients.Ophthalmic Epidemiol. 2004 Jul;11(3):241-53.

Personalised Health Management Systems
C.D. Nugent et al. (Eds.)
IOS Press, 2005

Context-Aware Infrastructure for Personalized Healthcare

Daqing ZHANG[1], Zhiwen YU[2], Chung-Yau CHIN[1]
[1]Context-Aware Systems Department, Institute for Infocomm Research,
21 Heng Mui Keng Terrace, Singapore 119613
[2]School of Computer Science, Northwestern Polytechnical University
Xi An, Shaan Xi, 710072, P.R. China

Abstract. Ubiquitous computing is shifting healthcare from treatment by professionals in hospitals to self-care, mobile care, home care and preventive care. In order to support the healthcare evolution, a global healthcare system, which links healthcare service providers to an individual's personal and physical spaces, is expected to provide personalized healthcare services at the right time, right place and right manner. This paper presents an overall architecture for such a context-aware healthcare system. The key technologies such as device self-sensing mechanism, context processing framework and a service interoperability platform are identified and elaborated. A personalized healthcare adviser service has been described to illustrate how personalized healthcare can be well supported by the proposed infrastructure.

Introduction

Today's paradigm of "one size fits all" healthcare is mainly applied in hospital, clinics and healthcare centers and is limited by the medical cost and resources. The emergence of ubiquitous computing and continuous progress in medical devices and diagnosis methodology, however, is enabling personalized healthcare services to be delivered to individuals at any place and any time. Personalized healthcare provides medical services which are truly effective "for me". This ensures that healthcare services provisioned to an individual are customized to his/her prevailing healthcare needs. With personalized healthcare, we can further achieve an "early health" system where disease is addressed and prevented at the earliest possible moment, rather than a "late disease" model where the emphasis is mainly on diagnosis and treatment.

To achieve healthcare personalization, without considering phenotypic and genotypic patient data, factors such as individual's lifestyle, surrounding situations, device capabilities, event of happenings, etc, should be taken into account. Such personalization factors are known as context, which refers to any information that can be used to characterize the situation of an entity (can be person, place or computational objects) and the interaction between them [1]. As a result, a personalized healthcare system is context-aware – provisioning healthcare information based on the user's changing context so that the right information can be delivered to the right person, at the right time, at the right place, using the right way.

In ubiquitous computing environments, computing entities ranging from sensors, actuators, devices to web services and applications, are supposed to scatter in different spaces and serve people even without their awareness. For example, a wearable health monitoring device can constantly examine one's blood pressure, body temperature, pulse, etc.; the availability of large display screen, surveillance camera and embedded microphone array at home may support remote medical consultation; web services can tell the consultation hours of a certain doctor. To fully exploit the power of the various hardware and software components, an infrastructure which enables device self-integration and service interoperability among heterogeneous functional components is required.

The objective of this paper is to present a scalable and flexible infrastructure for the delivery, management and deployment of context-aware personalized healthcare services to individuals via wide-area connectivity. Firstly, the key components of a global healthcare system are identified, then three enabling technologies to support such a global healthcare system are presented. Finally, a personalized healthcare adviser service is described to illustrate how personalized healthcare can be supported by the proposed architecture.

1. Global Healthcare System

The global healthcare system serves to provide a platform for managing and provisioning of healthcare services to individuals via the wide-area connectivity. It links the healthcare service providers to an individual's personal space, as well as physical smart spaces such as the home, car, office and school (see Figure 1). The key components can be grouped as follows:

Personal space is equipped with a network of wearable devices, sensors and digital equipment that can monitor an individual's health status and needs. An individual's personal space is enriched with context information, ranging from static information such as personal particulars, contact numbers, subscribed medical insurance and medical profile, to dynamic information such as health status, location and socializing record. It is important to collect such context information continuously as an individual makes the transition from a healthy state to illness and then on to recovery.

Smart space, on the other hand, is a physical environment where individual stay in. Despite the heterogeneity, it can react to the changes by dynamic reconfiguration and behaviour adaptation without user distraction. A smart space can be a house, hospital, vehicle, room, etc. With the proliferation of sensor techniques and information technologies, context information in a smart space is vastly available, ranging from low-level context (e.g. temperature, noise level, location coordinates, etc.) to high-level context (e.g. activity schedule, relations between individuals, event profile, etc).

Healthcare services are managed by the various independent healthcare service providers (e.g. physicians, professionals and caretakers) residing in remote spaces. Examples of healthcare services include medical consultation, emergency response, remote body check-up, insurance and billing. These services are supposed to adapt to the changing context of the service recipients.

Global Healthcare Network serves to link the personal spaces, smart spaces and healthcare service providers, providing a secure and reliable communication channel for services provisioning and context acquisition. An approach similar to [2] is adopted where a dynamic overlay network is constructed and maintained between the spaces, leveraging the Internet and the various wired (e.g. Ethernet, ADSL) and wireless (e.g. Wi-Fi, 3G, GPRS, Satellite) access network technologies.

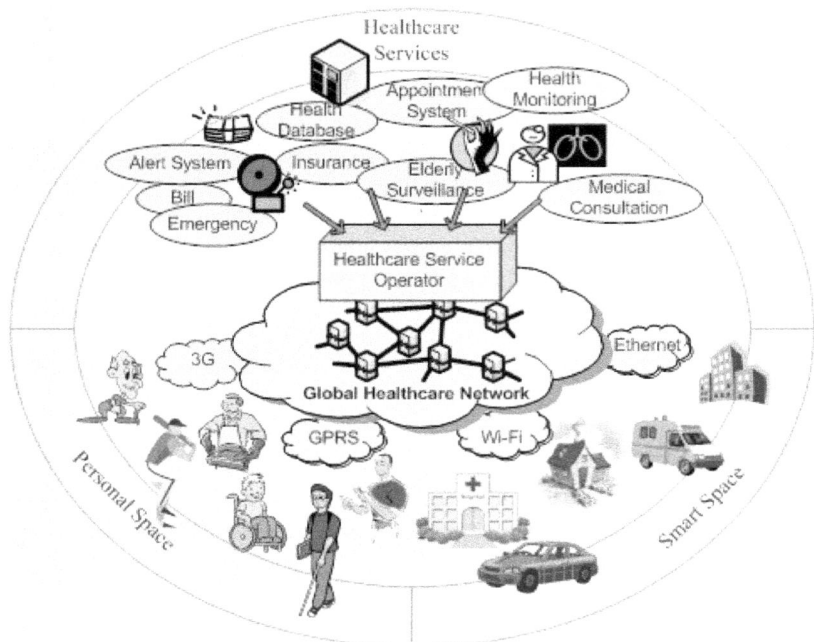

Figure 1. Global healthcare system overview.

The global healthcare system is composed of diverse spaces with various devices/services dynamically joining and leaving individual spaces. Both physical devices and software will offer certain kinds of services as a result. Together with the healthcare services provided by remote healthcare service providers, there is a need to interoperate these heterogeneous services for service management, delivery and composition. Services are composed and delivered to individuals based on the changing context. As context information is ubiquitously available in the personal and smart spaces, it needs to be aggregated, discovered, disseminated and interpreted for the healthcare service personalization process. To enable the healthcare system, infrastructure support addressing the issues of device, service and context is essentially required.

2. Enabling Technologies for Personalized Healthcare Infrastructure

To support rapid development and practical deployment of the context-aware personalized healthcare service in the global healthcare system, we require infrastructure support in terms of device access, context management, and service interoperability.

2.1. Device Access Mechanism

As the number of devices increases dramatically, device plug-and-play and self-integration features become critical. To minimize user intervention and support device interoperability, device self-configuration, discovery and proper capability announcement is highly desirable.

Each and every device in the personal space and smart space is equipped with self-sensing and self-configuration capability, which incorporates both capability publishing and capability discovering features. Capability publishing ensures a newly emerged device to announce its presence to the network, advertising its capability, resources and access information. The capability discovering feature, on the other hand, locates other devices in the network and makes use of the services provided by them. Universal Plug and Play (UPnP) [3] is an attempt towards device self-sensing and self-configuration. Further improvements need to be made to make devices self-integrated in the dynamic changing environment.

2.2. Context Management Framework

While the personal space and the smart space are enriched with a variety of heterogeneous context information, a common framework is needed to manage context. A context infrastructure is therefore proposed to handle context aggregation, discovery, inference and dissemination [4] (see Figure 2). The framework consists of the following components:

- **Context provider** is deployed to transform the raw context data into context mark-ups, providing an abstraction to separate the low-level sensing mechanism from the high-level context manipulation.
- **Context Aggregator** is responsible to gather and aggregate context mark-ups from the distributed context providers, and inserts them into the Context Knowledge Base.
- **Context Knowledge Base** (CKB) provides persistent context knowledge storage, and allows manipulation and retrieval by the Context Reasoner and Context Query Engine via proper interfaces.
- **Context Reasoner** infers high-level context information from basic sensed contexts using rule-based reasoning techniques, and also checks for knowledge consistency in the CKB.
- **Context Query Engine** (CQE) handles persistent queries and allows applications to extract desired context information from the CKB.
- **Context Discoverer** ensures the context requesters appropriately locate the components that can provide the desired and necessary context information. It

also supports wide-area context discovery across the local space boundaries [2].

- **Context-Aware Applications** utilize the high-level context information obtained from the CKB to adapt to rapidly changing situations. They can submit a persistent query to the CQE to ensure retrieval of the latest context information triggered by the context changes. To discover the relevant context information, the Context Discoverer can be relied on.

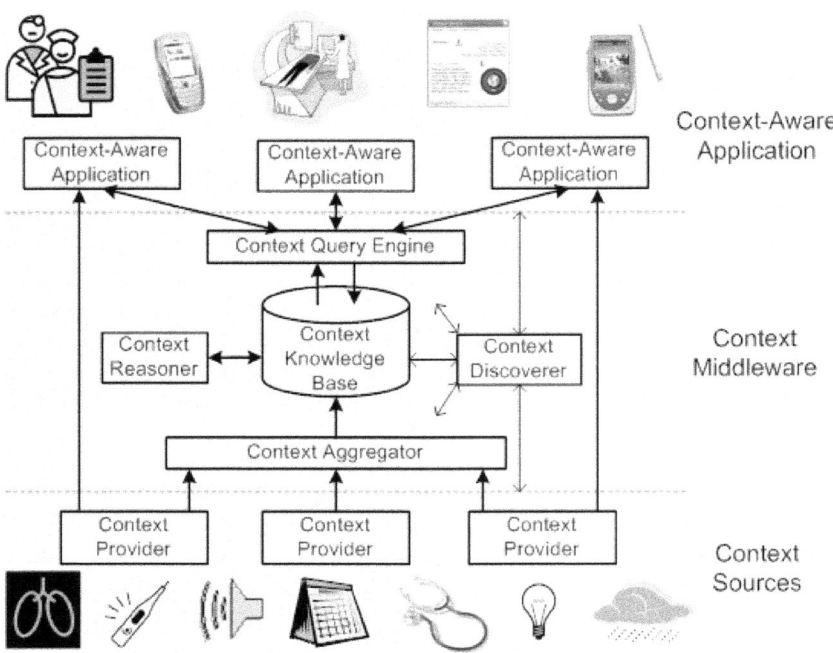

Figure 2. A layered context management framework.

2.3. Service Interoperability Platform

Healthcare services may vary in terms of their ability, vendor, access means and representation. To support service interoperability, we leverage service ontology as the representation model and service platform for managing and provisioning of services.

Ontology refers to the formal, explicit description of concepts, which are often conceived as a set of entities, relations, instances, functions and axioms [5]. With common ontological descriptions, the functionalities and relationship of devices, services and context could be machine-understandable at the semantics level. In such a way, devices can understand and collaborate with each other, context from diverse sources can be aggregated, and services can be easily deployed and composed.

Figure 3 shows the OSGi (Open Service Gateway Initiative) [6] based service delivery and management platform in the global healthcare system. The OSGi based service gateway is an open-standard based software framework enabling interoperability and co-existence of different services in a local space. It also facilitates secure and reliable provisioning of services to local-area environments via the wide-area network. The OSGi service framework provides a horizontal platform for hosting all kinds of service components, known as the *Service Bundle*, and interactions between bundles take place via the common bundle access APIs. As context management components and device access mechanisms can all be implemented in the form of service bundles together with other service functionalities, the OSGi platform provides a unified infrastructure to integrate the device, context and service, thus forms an ideal platform for personalized healthcare systems.

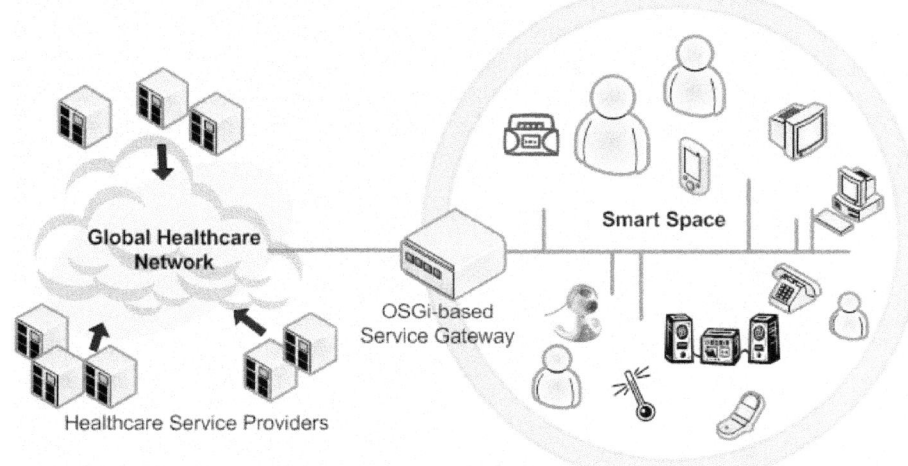

Figure 3. OSGi based service delivery and management platform.

3. Personalized Healthcare Adviser Service

Healthcare services, such as health monitoring, medical consultation, etc. need to be personalized based on context. We use here a personalized healthcare adviser service as a case study to illustrate how personalized healthcare is supported by the proposed infrastructure. The personalized healthcare adviser service provides health-related advice to the user in the right manner and at the right time.

For efficient processing of context in healthcare personalization, we classify the context into five categories: personal health context, environment context, task context, spatio-temporal context, and terminal context.

- **Personal health context** consists of two types: the physiological context and mental context. The former contains information like pulse, blood pressure, weight, glucose level, and retinal pattern. The latter includes context like mood, angriness, and stress etc.
- **Environment context** captures the entities that surround the users. These entities can be temperature, light, humidity, and noise.
- **Task context** describes the activities associated with the users. The task context can be described with explicit goals, tasks, actions, activities, or events.

- **Spatio-temporal context** refers to attributes like time and location.
- **Terminal context** is about the users' access network and devices. This includes information and attributes like: characteristics of the terminal (screen size, color quality of the screen, energy type, autonomy, OS, memory), interface (WIFI, Bluetooth, etc.), terminal type (PC, TV, PDA, STB, hand phone, etc.), media supported (audio, video, text, etc.).

Figure 4 shows the process for context-aware healthcare personalization. The key component is the personalization engine. It acquires different kinds of context from the context knowledge base, produces healthcare advice in an appropriate form, and delivers the healthcare service at the right time. The personalization engine leverages on the previous context infrastructure for context acquisition. The personalization engine consists of three elements: a healthcare advisor, a healthcare scheduler and a healthcare adapter.

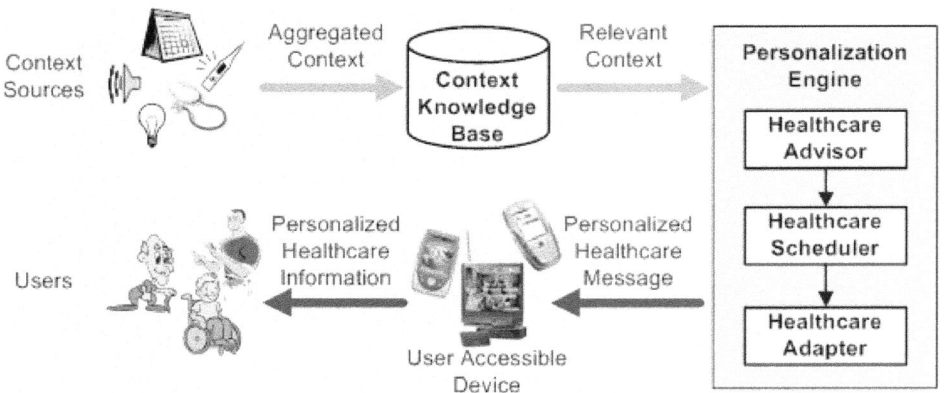

Figure 4. Context-aware healthcare personalization.

The healthcare advisor performs processing, reasoning, and behaviour analysis on the basis of a user's personal health context and/or environment context. It produces healthcare suggestions, such as a healthy lifestyle, diet and exercise. Healthcare suggestion may be, for example, "Your weight has increased too much in the last two days. You should eat more vegetables and do more exercise", "The office is too dry. The humidity generator should be turned on", etc.

The healthcare scheduler determines when to deliver advice to the user based on the user's current task context and/or spatio-temporal context. For instance, if the user is at an important meeting, the scheduler realizes that it is not a suitable time to send the message, and thus only informs the user later.

The healthcare adapter deals with the issue of how to present the service to the user. It performs content adaptation based on the terminal context, so that the user's accessible devices (PC, TV, PDA, hand phone, etc.) could present it and provide the best experience for the user. The content can be in the form of video, audio, image and text.

All of the healthcare advisor, scheduler, and adapter can work well by adopting rule-based techniques. Rule-based approaches determine which option should be taken in a specific situation by using a set of condition-actions rules. Each rule is an IF-THEN clause in nature. For example, the rules in Figure 5, infer personalized health advice based on the user's personal health context, deduce suitable delivering time based on the user's task context, and determine appropriate modality to present content based on terminal context. Such rules can be specified by healthcare experts or by a particular healthcare giver. They can also be obtained by using learning techniques the from user's behaviour or activity pattern.

IF weight/height exceeds a threthod, *THEN* do more exercise.

IF blood sugar exceeds a threthod, *THEN* should not take certain food.

IF the user is at meeting, *THEN* send the message later.

IF the user is at lunch, *THEN* send the message at once.

IF a PC is accessible, *THEN* present the message as video.

Figure 5. Sample rules.

We adopted first-order logic for reasoning about contexts. Forward chaining, backward chaining, and a hybrid execution model are supported. The forward-chaining rule engine is based on the standard Rete algorithm. The backward-chaining rule engine uses a logic-programming engine similar to Prolog engines. A hybrid execution mode performs reasoning by combining both forward and backward chaining. Our current system applies the Jena2 generic rule engine [7] to support forward-chaining reasoning over the context.

4. Related Work

In this section, we discuss related work in four areas: service platform, context middleware, personalization, and personalized healthcare.

Service platform. Several service platforms such as OSGi, Web service and .NET have been proposed to manage and provide healthcare services. While Web service and .NET are fully distributed service platforms, OSGi provides a centralized and hierarchical architecture for service provisioning and management. In particular, OSGi is designed to link the service providers with smart spaces via wide-area-network [8, 9] present an OSGi based service infrastructure for context-aware service in smart homes.

Context middleware. A few projects, including Context Toolkit [1], Semantic Space [4], UC Berkeley's open infrastructure [10], and the European Smart-Its project [11], specifically address the scalability and flexibility of context-aware applications by providing generic architectural supports. These projects generally provide infrastructure support for context-aware applications. They are not oriented towards healthcare services, and also lack personalization support.

Personalization. Personalization is about building customer loyalty by building a meaningful one-to-one relationship; by understanding the needs of each individual and helping satisfy a goal that efficiently and knowledgeably addresses each individual's need in a given context [12]. Personalization mainly consists of two steps: user modeling/profiling and content/service recommendation according to user profile. The recommendation techniques can be generally classified into rule-based, classifiers, clustering, and filtering-based methods. The filtering-based personalization systems provide recommendations based on user preference, which can be classified into content-based [13], collaborative [14], and hybrid methods [15].

Personalized healthcare. There has been some work performed in the area of personalized healthcare. Koutkias et al. [16] propose a system delivering personalized healthcare according to every patient's special requirements using the Wireless Application Protocol (WAP). This system involves monitoring and education services, designed specifically for people suffering from chronic diseases. It also applies data mining techniques to extract clinical patterns. Abidi et al. [17] introduce an intelligent Personalised Healthcare Information Delivery System that aims at enhancing patient empowerment by pro-actively pushing customised information, based on one's Electronic Medical Record and health maintenance information via the WWW. This system dynamically authors a HTML-based personalized health information package on the basis of an individual's current health profile. Takeshi et al. [18] developed health check-up services using mobile phones managing personal healthcare data in accordance with one's health awareness and lifestyle.

While few papers have addressed the infrastructure support for personalized healthcare in ubiquitous computing environments, this work attempts to identify the key components and enabling technologies for such an infrastructure. It is expected that personalized healthcare services can be provisioned at anytime, anywhere with the support of the infrastructure.

5. Conclusion

In this paper, we propose an infrastructure approach for context-aware healthcare personalization. The major contributions of the paper are: (1) identifying the logical components of a global healthcare system; (2) providing the enabling technologies for an infrastructure to support the global healthcare system in terms of device access, context management, and service interoperability; (3) illustrating how healthcare personalization is achieved by deploying the proposed infrastructure.

References

[1]   A.K. Dey, G. D. Abowd, D. Salber, "A Conceptual Framework and a Toolkit for Supporting the Rapid Prototyping of Context-Aware Applications", *Human-Computer Interaction (HCI) Journal*, 16(2-4), 2001.
[2]   D. Zhang, C. Y. Chin, M. Gurusamy, "Supporting Context-Aware Mobile Service Adaptation with Scalable Context Discovery Platform", To appear in *IEEE 61st Vehicular Technology Conference* (VTC2005-Spring).
[3]   Universal Plug and Play, http://www.upnp.org
[4]   X. Wang, D. Zhang, J. S. Dong, C. Y. Chin, and S. Hettiarachchi, "Semantic Space: An Infrastructure for Smart Spaces", *IEEE Pervasive Computing*, vol. 3, no. 3, 2004, pp. 32-39.
[5]   T. Gruber, "A Translation Approach to Portable Ontology Specification," Knowledge Acquisition, Vol. 5, No. 2, 1993, pp. 199-220.
[6]   Open Service Gateway initiative (OSGi), http://www.osgi.org
[7]   J.J. Carroll, et al., "Jena: Implementing the Semantic Web Recommendations", *Proc. of 13th Intl Conf. on World Wide Web*. New York. 2004.
[8]   Daqing Zhang, et al. "OSGi Based Service Infrastructure for Context Aware Connected Homes". *1st International Conference on Smart Homes and Health Telematics* (ICOST2003), Sep. 24, 2003, France.

[9] Sumi Helal, et al. "Smart Phone Based Cognitive Assistant". *The 2nd International Workshop on Ubiquitous Computing for Pervasive Healthcare Applications* (UbiHealth2003), October 12, 2003.

[10] J.I. Hong and J.A. Landay "An Infrastructure Approach to Context-Aware Computing", *Human-Computer Interaction*, vol. 16, nos. 2-4, 2001, p. 97.

[11] H. Gellersen et al., "Physical Prototyping with Smart-Its", *IEEE Pervasive Computing*, vol. 3, no. 3, 2004, pp. 74-82.

[12] Doug Riecken, "Personlized Views of Personalization", *Communications of the ACM*, vol. 43, no. 8, 2000

[13] Zhiwen Yu and Xingshe Zhou. "TV3P: An Adaptive Assistant for Personalized TV". *IEEE Transactions on Consumer Electronics*. Vol. 50, No. 1, 2004, pp. 393-399

[14] Resnick, P., et al. "GroupLens: An open architecture for collaborative filtering of netnews". In *Proc. Of 1994 Computer Supported Cooperative Work Conference*.

[15] N. Good, et al. "Combining collaborative filtering with personal agents for better recommendations". *Proc. Of 1999 Conf. of the AAAI*.

[16] V. G. Koutkias, S. L. Meletiadis, and N, Maglaveras, "WAP-based personalized healthcare system", *Health Informatics Journal*, Vol. 7, No. 3-4, pp.183-189, 2001

[17] S.S.R. Abidi and A. Goh, "A personalised Healthcare Information Delivery System: pushing customised healthcare information over the WWW", *Medical Infobahn in Europe* (MIE2000), IOS Press, Amsterdam

[18] Takeshi Hashiguchi, Hitoshi Matsuo, and Akihide Hashizume, "Healthcare Dynamics Informatics for Personalized Healthcare", *Hitachi Review* Vol. 52, No. 4, pp. 183-188, 2003

Personalised Health Management Systems
C.D. Nugent et al. (Eds.)
IOS Press, 2005

Software and Knowledge Engineering Aspects of Smart Homes Applied to Health

Juan Carlos AUGUSTO[1], Chris NUGENT[1], Suzanne MARTIN[2], Colin OLPHERT[1]
[1] School of Computing and Mathematics, Faculty of Engineering
[2] School of Health Sciences, Faculty of Life and Health Science
University of Ulster at Jordanstown, UK

Abstract. Smart Home technology offers a viable solution to the increasing needs of the elderly, special needs and home based-healthcare populations. The research to date has largely focused on the development of communication technologies, sensor technologies and intelligent user interfaces.

We claim that this technological evolution has not been matched with a step of a similar size on the software counterpart. We particularly focus on the software that emphasizes the intelligent aspects of a Smart Home and the difficulties that arise from the computational analysis of the information collected from a Smart Home. The process of translating information into accurate diagnosis when using non-invasive technology is full of challenges, some of which have been considered in the literature to some extent but as yet without clear landmarks.

Keywords. Smart Homes, intelligent environments, home healthcare, personalization.

Introduction

The application of Smart Home technology is used to enhance the quality of life of elderly people and in particular to those experiencing some degree of cognitive impairment (e.g., early dementia symptoms) [1, 2]. The rationale for the Smart Home is founded on the potential of Information and Communications Technology (ICT) to support independent living and extend the period of time a person can remain in their own home when integrated into a Social Care model [3]. From a European perspective, the European Commission considers that ICT integrated into healthcare has a strong and positive role to play [4].

The underlying technology within the Smart Home environment comprises of three main components: communications, computing and user interfaces. A variety of studies have been reported deploying each of these as a means to support independent living. Examples range from social alarms to healthcare monitoring to interaction with various home appliances [5, 6]. Nevertheless, it is apparent that within this area the majority of the focus has been towards the provision of the technology within the home as opposed to the analysis of the information generated and the application of these results to proactively change the living experience and inform service providers, so enabling scarce care resources to be effectively targeted towards specific needs.

The focus of our current study relates to the integration of Artificial Intelligence and Software Engineering techniques with the social aspects (health priorities and aims, interaction with carers, etc.) derived from the environment where Smart Home technology is applied. Within this context we focus on the intelligent analysis of the information gathered through sensors and apply spatio-temporal reasoning to define a monitoring system and anticipate situations of interest for example when the person may be in danger or when they may experience a form of discomfort. From a holistic perspective, the application of this technology supports the idea that, for a Smart Home system to be effective for our society, the technology inside the Smart Home has to be linked to the surrounding environment in the health care system where it is applied and with those who are providing care for the dependant person.

This vision can be achieved by providing a link between the lifestyle related information gathered by the system and the carers who provide support for the person in their home. This will allow each of these elements to interact and inform each other in a natural and fluent way.

1. Smart Home Environment

For this work we are adopting a Smart Home framework which has been proposed elsewhere [7, 8]. In this scenario it is assumed that the house itself is equipped with a number of sensors for monitoring purposes. Examples of these include sensors to monitor risk situations (Fire alarms, Smoke alarms, Emergency pull cord, Anti burglar alarm), to monitor activities (Movement detectors, Door ID tag detector, Pressure mats, Water tap sensors, Cooker sensor) and to facilitate medication management. In this environment, the activation or the inclusion of the sensors within a given person's home depends upon their current health status and the 'risks', based on this status, which are likely to occur. Other parameters such as levels of privacy and caring infrastructure can be tailored and agreed between the caring personnel and the beneficiaries.

Spatio-temporal reasoning is a core component of the real-time monitoring system. Sensors within the home environment provide information relating to the person's activities. This information relates to firstly their whereabouts, and secondly their interaction with appliances. It is important when considering this information to give an appreciation for the ordering of different events and in addition the time which has elapsed between them. This is necessary in order for an assessment of the current situation of the dependant to be made and to distinguish between a range of options for example 'hazardous', 'potentially hazardous', 'requiring communication with person', 'non-hazardous', etc. [9].

The monitoring system is based on a blend of technologies. At its core, an Active Database (ADB) framework centred on ECA (Event-Condition-Action) rules is used to capture events occurring in meaningful contexts. The general schema for ECA rules is shown in Figure 1 along with an example of how it can be used in this context.

ON *<event expression>*	ON "cooker has been turned on in the past"
	and "dependant person leaves kitchen"
IF *<condition>*	IF "dependant person goes to bed for a 'long' period of time"
THEN *<action>*	THEN "turn cooker off" and "notify carers"

Figure 1. ECA rule construct: general scheme and example of its usage.

Space restrictions limit the technical details which can be presented. Further details can be found in [7]. The ADB system is only a part of the entire system architecture which involves different layers ranging from the human-computer interfaces to the sensors operating inside the Smart Home (see [8] for details of the complete system architecture.)

A graphical representation of the Smart Home has been developed to act as an interface between the underpinning ADB and the carer monitoring the activities of the person within their home environment. This consists of a map of the Smart Home and a marker which represents the (dependant) person within the home environment. Messages are displayed below the map indicating a log of activities and warning messages are presented to the carer in instances of potentially hazardous situations. From an operational perspective the interface supports the presentation of two different levels of activities of the person. In the first instance, movement is presented as the marker moves through the varying rooms according to the movement of the person as detected by the motion sensors. Secondly, as the person interacts with various appliances equipped with sensors for example the cooker, the bed or taps, these are highlighted to indicate a level of interaction. In addition to visual warning messages in potentially hazardous situations the interface also provides an audible alert. Carers, upon receiving a warning, have the choice to summon assistance for the resident or dismiss the warning using their own judgment.

Figure 2 below shows the reaction from the system under the conditions represented in Figure 1. This shows how the interface has the ability to represent the person's movement within the home environment and also their interaction with appliances. (Only snapshots are presented here. Whilst running in real time the person's movement is represented by a dot moving throughout the interface.) Figure 2 (a) provides initial information indicating that the person is located in the bedroom. In Figure 2 (b) the person has moved from the bedroom to the kitchen and has turned the cooker on. In Figure 2 (c) the person has returned to the bedroom and the bed sensor has detected the person is now lying down. After a predefined interval of time the system, based on the aforementioned ECA rule schema has inferred this situation to be one which should be considered as potentially hazardous and subsequently informed the interface to provide an alarm message.

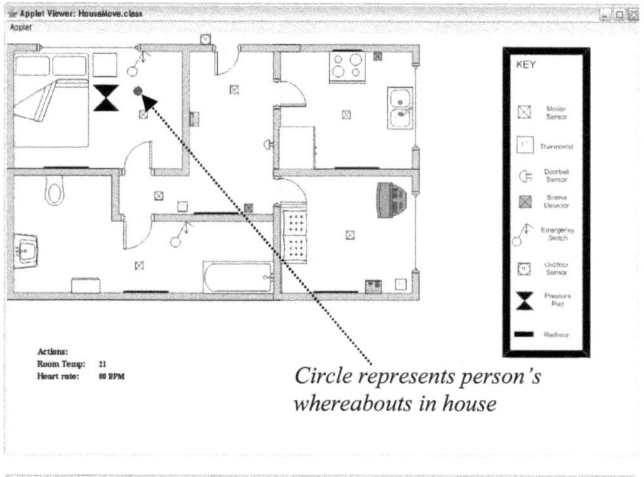

a) At this point the person is in the bedroom as represented by the small dot/circle.

Circle represents person's whereabouts in house

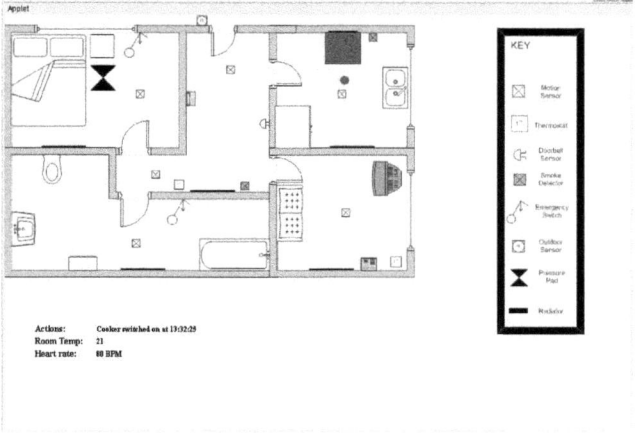

b) The person has moved to the kitchen and turned on the cooker.

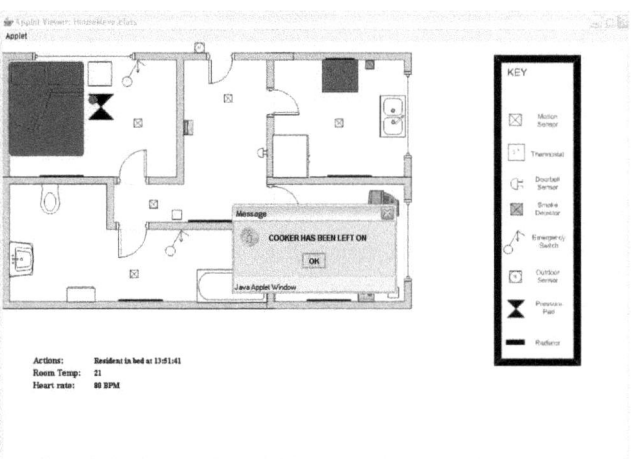

c) The person has returned to the bedroom and entered the bed. The system has reacted accordingly after a fixed unit of time by indicating a potentially hazardous situation and providing a warning message.

Figure 2. Scenarios of monitoring system. (a) Person in bedroom (b) person in kitchen and turned cooker on (c) person in bed and alarm raised as cooker is still on.

2. Integrated Service Model – Future Vision

The system we are proposing provides two main services. Firstly it monitors a person and reacts accordingly in real-time in situations of concern as previously described in Section 2. Secondly it provides a longer-term interaction with the person's healthcare care plan by recording all of their activities and providing sufficient information for lifestyle profiling. It is this long term interaction that forms our visionary concepts for the further developments within this arena to provide an enhanced level of support to the person and also the carers who support them.

Key to these developments is the care plan which is stored for each person in such an environment. Care plans contain sets of instructions and health related information describing the healthcare needs and the levels of support required. By considering this information in conjunction with the long term activity profiles of the person, recorded by the Smart Home, offers two advantages:

- An assessment can be made relating to how well synchronized the deployment of the system is with respect to the details of the care plan.
- Changes in the care plan based on lifestyle changes may be possible.

Figure 3 below shows an overview of this vision. At the centre of the system is the person within the home environment. By recording information over a long period of time profiles can be produced relating to the person's activities within the home, their pattern of movements and their interaction with appliances. Our vision is that this information can be somehow analysed to provide an indication of lifestyle patterns. Information from this can then be used to update the care plan to offer improved levels of care as the lifestyles and hence needs of the person changes.

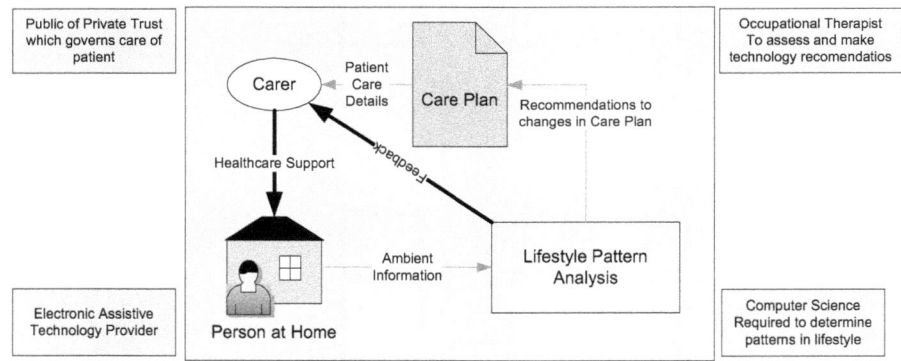

Figure 3. An Integrated Service Model interacting with the care plan.

To gain an appreciation as to the exact extent to which the care plan can be modified requires a closer examination of its content. Sections of a typical care plan of particular importance from our perspective are: "needs assessment", "incident reporting", and "dependant/carer care plan":

- "needs assessment" - this relates to the individual special needs (hearing impairment, medication requirements, physical and cognitive abilities).
- "dependant/carer care plan" - this provides valuable information relating to: Hygienic/social/spiritual/dietary routines, staff rota and agreed call times

when carers will visit the person in their home to provide a form of predefined healthcare assistance.

- "incident reporting" – the outcome of the carers' activities are usually recorded and if special actions were taken following a particular incident they must be logged.

It is our goal to map the information within the care plan, in the first instance, to the rule base which governs the decision support mechanism for determining situations of potential concern. In essence this relates to the schemas which must be established in the production of the ECA rules. For example, from the "needs assessment" we can extract:

- which are the events the system must focus on for a particular individual and
- the contexts where risk factors are relevant

From the "dependant/carer care plan" we can extract:

- How can the house be accessed?
- Who can access the house?
- When is it more appropriate to be visited, if a choice is possible?

The information included in a person's "needs assessment" is clearly related to the Events and Conditions parts of the ECA rules (refer to Figure 1 above) whilst the care plan details information on how the caring environment should react to an incident, i.e., the Actions part of the ECA rules. Once the information transfer from the care plan to the ECA rule schema has been established it provides the potential opportunity to asses the lifestyle patterns of the person over time and subsequently make recommendations as to how the care plan should be changed to accommodate these patterns. Figure 4 shows how the lifestyle monitoring can be included with the ADB at the core of the system.

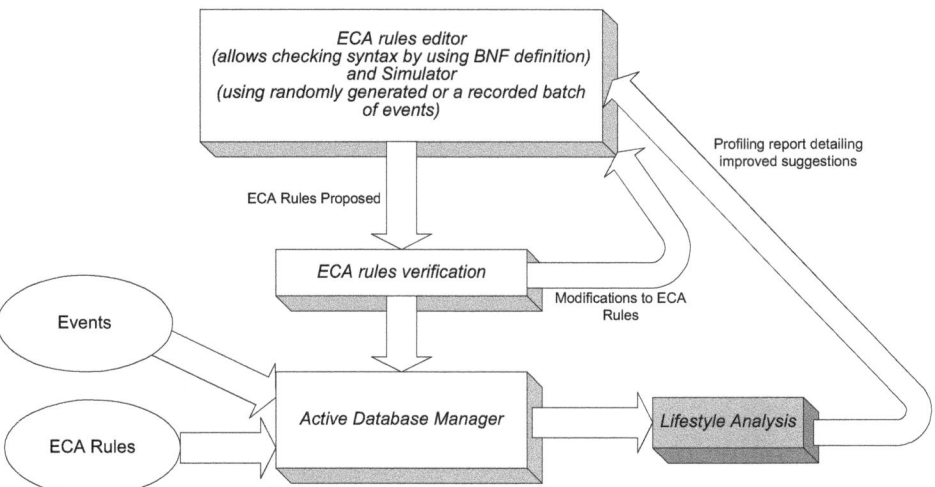

Figure 4. Incorporation of lifestyle analysis in overall software infrastructure.

Over a period of time a profile can be constructed of the person by logging all of their daily activities. Such a profile can contain valuable information showing trends in a person's lifestyle and more importantly how these trends deviate from the initial care plan which has been established.

From a computational perspective statistical analyses and software-based learning mechanisms can be used to detect when deviations from the expected care plan occur. Discovery techniques, e.g. Data Mining, can be introduced to discover new emerging patterns of behaviour not considered, nor accommodated, by the current static care plan. For example, cognitive deterioration can cause the dependant person to start loosing the sense of time (e.g., reversing day/night activities). Alternatively, during the winter months a person may chose to remain in bed for a longer period of time in the mornings, hence alarms based around a specified time, after which an alarm should be raised if the dependant person has been detected as still being in bed, should be modified.

Detections in changes of lifestyle should then be used to change the care plan on a person-per-person basis hence offering a level of individual personalisation of Smart Home support. Information detailing the changes required should be presented by the system in two means. In the first instance, feedback from the system should be presented to the carers indicating how improved healthcare services could be provided. At this stage the system should allow them to directly adjust the care plan (e.g. increasing/reducing visits/medicine). This will in effect result in modifications being made to the ECA schemas. In the second instance, were modifications to the system are quantitative in nature, for example changing the time of the first home visit of the day, automatic changes to the care plan and form of healthcare delivery can be made.

3. Conclusions

Care plans are a rich source of information on how care should be provided to the person and within the Smart Home environment, how the system is expected to run. We have considered the need for intelligent analysis of data in Smart Homes to increase personal autonomy and re-incorporation into society of elderly people with cognitive impairment. This article stresses the fact that Smart Home systems operate within a community and hence the importance of exercising the two directions relating to the flow of information between the software infrastructure layer and the surrounding traditional healthcare system.

On one hand the system gives the carers advice on the long-term functionality of the monitoring process and events which frequently caused concerns. On the other hand it facilitates the participation of carers in the functionality of the system so that they suggest alterations to the system reflecting changes to be made to the care plan. Naturally, not all of the process is automatic. Part of our current work is devoted to discern where the line between the automatic and the manual modifications to the care plan has to be drawn for this particular project.

Our vision is one which extends the notion of a Smart Home by making use of the valuable information which can be recorded by all of the sensing technology and conveying this to caring staff through communications infrastructures. Our vision is to provide a truly personalized healthcare service by adapting the technological and human care support offered to the evolving lifestyle patterns of the citizen. We believe our vision can be achieved with the technical concepts presented.

References

[1] *Independent living for persons with disabilities and elderly people Proceedings of 1st International Conference on Smart Homes and Health Telematics (ICOST'2003).* Assistive Technology Research Series, Volume 12. M. Mokhtari Ed., Paris, 2003.

[2] *Toward a Human Friendly Assistive Environment (Proceedings of 2nd International Conference On Smart homes and health Telematic, ICOST2004).* Assistive Technology Research Series, Volume 14, IOS Press, D. Zhang and M. Moktari Eds., Singapore, September 15-17, 2004.

[3] G.   Dewsbury, B. Taylor,. M. Edge (2001) *Designing safe smart home systems for Vulnerable people* in Dependability in Healthcare informatics, R Proctor and M Rouncefield eds, Proceedings of the first Dependability IRC Workshop, Edinburgh March 22-23 Lancaster University.

[4] European Commission (2004). eHealth – making healthcare better for European Citizens: An action plan for a European eHealth Area. (SEC(2004)539).

[5] S. Helal (2003). Assistive environments for successful aging. In M. Mokhatari (Ed*) Independent living for Persons with Disabilities and Elderly People*, IOS press.

[6] M.J. Fisk (2003) *Social Alarms to Telecare. Older People's Services in Transition.* Bristol: Policy Press.

[7] J.C. Augusto and C. D. Nugent The Use of Temporal Reasoning and Management of Complex Events in Smart Homes.. Proceedings of European Conference on Artificial Intelligence (ECAI 2004), edited by R. López de Mántaras and L. Saitta, IOS Press (Amsterdam, The Netherlands), pp. 778-782, held in Valencia, Spain, August 22-27, 2004.

[8] J. C. Augusto and C. D. Nugent. A New Architecture for Smart Homes Based on ADB and Temporal Reasoning.. In "Toward a Human Friendly Assistive Environment" (Proceedings of 2nd International Conference On Smart homes and health Telematic, ICOST2004), Assistive Technology Research Series, Vol. 14, pp. 106-113, D. Zhang, M. Mokhtari eds., IOS Press, Singapore, Sept. 15-17, 2004.

[9] C. D. Nugent and J. C. Augusto. Management and Analysis of Time-Related Data in Internet Based Healthcare Delivery. To be published in "Clinical Knowledge Management", edited by R. Bali, Idea Group Publishing, USA. 2005.

Personalised Health Management Systems
C.D. Nugent et al. (Eds.)
IOS Press, 2005

End-to-End Signal Processing from the Embedded Body Sensor to the Medical End User Through QoS-Less Public Communication Channels: The U-R-SAFE Experience

Francis CASTANIE, Corinne MAILHES, Stéphane HENRION
ENSEEIHT-IRIT-TéSA, 2 rue Camichel, BP7122, 31071 Toulouse Cédex 7, France

Abstract. The URSafe project (IST-2001-33352) aims at creating a telemedicine care environment for the elderly and convalescent. The idea is to provide a portable device which monitors autonomously different biomedical signals and is able to send an alarm to a medical center if an abnormality is detected. In the initial version of URSafe, three sensors where included in the platform: electrocardiogram (ECG), oxygen rate (SpO2) and Fall Detector. This paper presents the signal processing algorithms involved in the project. These are at two levels : ECG analysis and signal transmission.

Keywords. ECG analysis, Pathology detection, lost sample recovering.

Introduction

Chronic conditions are becoming the first problem of public health in Western countries. The URSAFE project (http://ursafe.tesa.prd.fr) has been proposed within this field. It includes sensors (ECG, Oxygen saturation and fall detection) that monitor the patient's condition. All are linked to a central unit, called a Portable Base Station (PBS), through Ultra Wide Band (UWB) techniques. Alarm management is implemented at each sensor level. Dealing with oxygen saturation and fall detection, these are very simple. Regarding ECG analysis, the aim of URSAFE is to provide a detector for pathological condition warning and, if possible, a pre-diagnosis for this condition identification. The field of applications of the URSAFE objectives concerns 6 classes of pathologies: tachycardia, bradycardia, atrial fibrillation, ventricular fibrillation, ventricular tachycardia and atrial-ventricular block. The first part of this paper presents the signal processing algorithms developed for these abnormality detections.

When an alarm is detected at the monitoring device level, a transmission scenario through the complete communication link (terrestrial or satellite, depending on the availability) is initiated. It includes the warning of a medical center through the transmission of a few minutes of patient recorded biomedical data. Once those data are received, a medical expert may analyze the data, to confirm the diagnosis made at the patient level (monitoring device level) and eventually activate an emergency situation.

Therefore the quality of the received data for the medical expert is very important to provide an efficient solution. As the transmission uses a wide variety of communication links, errors are likely to occur along the transmission chain. In the second part of the paper an approach to ensure medically-readable information through protection (coding) means and an associated restoration process is presented.

1. Electrocardiogram (ECG) Analysis

The aim of the signal processing algorithms implanted in the URSAFE system has two distinct objectives :

The first objective is to **detect** a pathology through the continuous analysis of the recorded biomedical signal (ECG), including beat detection (QRS location) and beat identification (beat feature extraction and analysis).

The second objective is to **perform a pre-diagnosis** for the identification of the warned condition.

A general overview of the existing approaches to tackle the QRS detection is proposed in [1]. Well-known and widely validated QRS detection algorithms are easy to implement, based on a first stage of filtering used to enhance a specific feature in the ECG signal, followed by a threshold detection procedure with the enhanced feature. A generic review of such algorithms is proposed in [2]. All are based on QRS amplitude or derivative (or combined) feature considerations. The main advantage is their computing simplicity, and many of them provide good results, such as the well known *"Pan-Tompkins"* algorithm [3].

Within the frame of the URSAFE project, the processor included in the ECG sensor is a micro controller (Hitachi H8S/2655). Therefore, due to computational costs, the chosen QRS detection algorithm is the Pan-Tompkins one.

Once the QRS complex location is estimated, some additional processing modules are required at the output of the detector to correctly locate the R wave, that will additionally provide a precise estimation of the R-R interval as well as the HRV (Heart Rate Variability). This allows the estimation of the QRS width, as well as the P wave detection based on [4]. In [4], noise corrupted abrupt changes are detected with the use of a continuous time scale analysis. In order to detect the P wave, different detectors have been tested (based either on correlation max or correlation sum over scales and using different wavelet types). The best results have been obtained with a detector based on the measure of similarity between a continuous wavelet transform of a signature and of the current analysed segment likely to contain a P wave. The signature is the first derivation of a Gaussian waveform (close to the shape of a P wave). Then its continuous wavelet transform using the "mexican hat" is computed over the scales 1 to 10. Thus, a 2D (time and scale) map of the continuous wavelet transform is obtained. A similar map for the first derivative of the analysed segment is also computed.

Different detection criteria have been studied. The most promising seems to be the one that sums over the scales of the temporal cross correlation of the two previous maps. A threshold level was set with a tested P wave database (extracted from the MIT BIH signals).

Once the QRS location and some features obtained either at mid term (beats sequence) level (RR statistics) or at beat level (QRS width, PR interval) are known, we have to classify the current beat. This part of the algorithm is the most critical of the whole detector. Its organisation tries to follow the expert's way of thinking (knowledge and uncertainty) about the diagnosis and according to the field of our software. It is mainly based on IF-THEN fuzzy rules and has been designed jointly with a medical expert. Moreover, validation of the whole detector has been tested on ECG signals from the MIT-BIH data base and results have been compared to the medical expert provided by a cardiologist on the same signals.

2. ECG Transmission

The URSafe scenario includes the transmission of the last minute of the recorded ECG to the medical centre for expert analysis when an abnormality is detected.

According to the different characteristics of the transmission channels (bandwidth, memory storage capability) likely to be used between the sensor and the medical center, some additional signal processing may be required. This is mainly due to channel transmission bit rate capabilities (compression) and channel error models (coding and restoration) that could lead to partial data losses.

The different links (fixed access network (PSTN), mobile access network (GSM/GPRS and future UMTS) or satellite interfacing (DVB-RCS technology)) included in this transmission chain are likely to induce errors on the transmitted data. These errors/losses can occur anytime and anywhere (according to the channel availability, memory overflows, protocol....) during a transmission process and can only be assessed in a statistical way. Indeed a fixed Quality of Service (QoS) does exist only if an end-to-end connection is reserved for the application. But this is not the case for the URSAFE project, which uses public networks between the local PBS and the medical center.

As no connectionless transmission is able to provide null error rates, when a quantified QoS cannot be ensured, the common way of obtaining the desired data when a transmission error is stated (through error detection coding) is the use of a retransmission process. The receiver notices the transmission error and asks for the re-sending of the data. But whatever the retransmission process (ARQ protocol) of the different layers of the protocols (either TCP in the IP scenario, or in 3 different sub-layers in GPRS), there is no way to provide null error rates (except if an infinite transmission delay is acceptable). According to the medical application of the URSAFE concept, the maximum acceptable delay has been stated.

This first version of the URSAFE concept is not dedicated to emergency cases (no information about the patient location is included in the system). But in future developments of the system, more restriction about the transmission delay will be required for an efficient emergency service provision.

Thus we can sum up the transmission chain (and its specificity) in the URSAFE concept concerning the ECG data (the longest to transmit) in two segments of 30 seconds each (before and after alarm event setting).

When a complete ECG message of 30 seconds length has been received at the PBS, the transmission to the medical center is initiated. One of the three possible networks is selected by the PBS. The data binary message length is organized in packets and transmitted on the selected network which uses a specific protocol.

If some errors (packet losses) are detected in the different layers of the data exchange protocol, then retransmission processes take place (based on the multiple retransmission ARQ protocol(s)), introducing delays in the global message transmission. It is not generally possible to intervene at the sub-layer level to modify the ARQ processes and thus to stop the multiple retransmissions. Thus according to the medical side, a *time out point* is defined, which is the maximum time delay until we consider the associated packet as lost. At the Medical Center level, due to the use of an error detection code (CRC) on the transmitted binary data, we are able to know which packet is missing or lost and which packet is missing according to the *time out* delay.

Thus from the signal processing point of view, we can only base our approach on statistics of the missing packets, that is to say the packet loss probability. It may be possible to have this statistic as a function of the retransmission delay. Packet loss does occur over GPRS links in both the downlink and up-link directions, but the incidence is relatively rare, and hard to quantify. When loss does occur, it is quite likely to occur in bursts of consecutive packets. As a general guideline, in core network design the packet loss probability is ideally set to 1% (however in real life can vary between 1-2% dependent on CDMA, FDMA, TDMA schemes and the factor mentioned above). Using satellite links, this probability can grow up to 8%.

2.1. Strategy and Solutions to Overcome the Transmissions Losses

A defined QoS exists only if an end-to-end connection is reserved for the application and this is not the case for URSAFE. Therefore, a strategy has to be decided. At the end user side, the medical doctor can receive data (ECG signals, mainly) with some possible "holes" in it, due to packet losses. The length of the missing samples is a direct function of the length of lost packets.

Two possibilities can occur:

- Either these packets arrive within an acceptable delay and the display is updated,
- Or these packets do not arrived after a maximum acceptable delay (acceptable for the medical end user).

In this last case, some restoration algorithms can be used in order to propose a way to restore the missing segments in the ECG display. Obviously, these restored samples will be highlighted (or displayed in a different color) in order for the medical doctor to be aware of the portions of the ECG which have been restored. As soon as the missing packets arrive at the end user side, the restored samples will be replaced by the real data.

2.2. State of the Art of Restoration Scheme

The reconstruction of partially known signals has been widely studied in the signal processing literature. A very good review can be found in [5]. Deeper studies can be found in [6] and [7]. In these papers, it is assumed that the signals are partially known in the sense that only a subset of its samples is supposed to be available for measurement. The problem is then to determine the signal from the available samples.

The constraint extensively used in recovery of missing samples is the frequency band-limitation. In the case of ECG signals, sampled at 250 Hz, this constraint can be considered. Clearly, ECG signals can be assumed to be band-limited between 1 and 30 Hz. This band-limitation condition allows the problem of recovering lost samples not to be ill-posed. Therefore, a trivial necessary condition is that the remaining number of samples (without those being lost) should be at least equal to *2M+1*, i.e. the dimension of the subspace of the low-pass signal *x*. For ECG signals, *M* is such that:

$$M = \frac{30}{250} N = 0.12N$$

Therefore, the above condition on the ECG is that it remains at least 24% of the samples. But note immediately that this represents a theoretical minimum condition. In practice, it is obvious that the efficiency of missing sample recovery algorithms will highly depend on how the missing samples are distributed over the total *N* samples. The worst case is when the missing samples are contiguous, as in the case of extrapolation problems. Scattered missing data usually leads to well-posed and stable reconstruction problems, whereas extrapolation leads to ill-posed, numerically difficult problems. In simulations and validations of the proposed algorithms, we have considered the worst case, i.e. the case where the missing samples are contiguous. But, it is important to note that the same reconstruction algorithms can be used in the case of scattered missing data with better results. Therefore, it will be interesting to propose a packet formation for ECG transmission in order to minimize the probability of missing samples to be contiguous (see section *2.5*).

2.3. Lost Sample Recovering Algorithms

The historical method proposed for the missing data problem is the Papoulis-Gerchberg (P-G) algorithm [6]. This is an iterative method, each iteration being based on a two-step procedure : filtering and re-sampling.

The main interest of this algorithm is its computational cost, based on the Fast Fourier Transform (FFT) algorithm. However, the main drawback of the P-G algorithm lies in its convergence rate. When the missing sample number is small, a few iterations are necessary to obtain a quasi-perfect result. However, the results of the P-G algorithm are less impressive when the number of missing samples is more important.

However, a more general algorithm has been proposed, linked to constrained iterative restoration [6], by introducing a relaxation factor, μ, in the P-G algorithm. In order to optimize the convergence rate of the algorithm, the value of μ can be computed. However, whenever there are long contiguous gaps of missing samples, the convergence rate falls down to very low values.

A third class of restoration algorithms has been proposed which performs better than P-G based algorithms. These are based on the minimum dimension method [6].

The main point of interest with the minimum dimension method is that it leads to sets of linear equations for the unknown samples, with as many equations as unknown samples, thus with a lower computational cost than P-G algorithms. The second and final point of interest with this class of algorithm is that results on ECG signals are more promising.

2.4. Results on ECG Restoration

Although ECGs are band-limited signals, they are non-stationary which may degrade the proposed algorithm's performance. Moreover, restoration algorithm results may highly depend on the *position* of the missing samples. Therefore, all proposed algorithms have been tested on portions of 512 points of ECG signals and for different localizations of the missing samples.

Results show that a maximum 1% of 2% of contiguous missing samples can be recovered using the P-G algorithm. Note that if the missing samples were not contiguous, obviously, the percentage of missing samples which can be recovered by this algorithm would be higher.

The constrained iterative restoration algorithm which belongs to the same class of algorithms as the P-G algorithms gives similar results on ECG signals. Note that the computing cost of optimum relaxation factor may be a strong drawback of this algorithm, since the restoration algorithms are used while the end user system will wait for the lost packet to arrive.

The last proposed algorithm, the minimum dimension formulation, performs very well on ECG signals, using some modification (pre-filtering with an ideal filter at the assumed cut frequency, here, 30 Hz). The problems of ill-conditioned matrix appear for a number of contiguous missing samples exceeding 45 (over 512). This seems a value above which the transmission problem should not exist. However, if error propagation studies lead to consider that such a percentage of contiguous missing samples can have a non-negligible probability, solutions exist, by implementing sophisticated algorithms for linear system solving.

What is more important, is that the results given by this algorithm are far better than the one obtained with the P-G based algorithm. First, the evolution of the restoration error power as a function of the number of missing samples does not depend on the position of these missing samples, as was observed for the P-G algorithm. Whatever the position, the error power is the same and is less than that with the P-G algorithm and allows considering that *a maximum of 40 contiguous missing samples can be recovered (over 256)*. Figure 1 presents a restoration example.

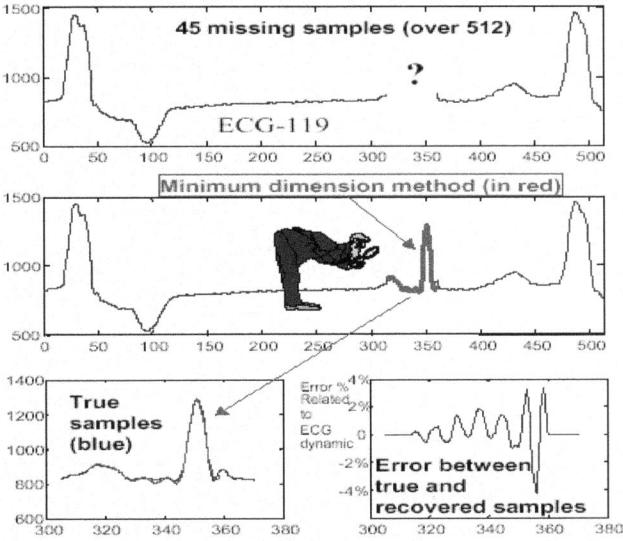

Figure. 1 : Example of ECG sample recovering.

2.5. Data Organization to be Compliant with the Restoration Capabilities

From the previous results, at the end user level, the restoration process is able to restore 40 successive missing samples within a window width of 256 samples. As the data are basically coded in 10bits, this allows a loss of 400 bits or 50 bytes.

Therefore the maximum data message length to transmit in the URSAFE project (without compression) is 75Kbits or 9.375Kbytes (30 seconds of recorded ECG). Thus the maximum data length likely to be lost is around 200 bytes !

Consequently it is necessary to consider a specific data organization prior to transmission. Thus, we propose to divide the total message length (30seconds of ECG) in blocks of K temporal samples. Then an interleaving code of these blocks is performed before binary packing and transmission (M blocks in a packet). According to the maximum data length restoration capability, (40 per section), the block sizing can be considered between 1 and 40 samples.

The aim of the interleaving is to ensure that the resulting "holes" (in the recovered signal) have a length below 40 samples and are separated by at least 256 samples, according to the restoration capabilities. For this purpose, we have studied the compromise on block length, packet size and spacing between two consecutive blocks in the interleaving coded message. For our application, one good compromise seems to be the following interleaving scheme :
-   a block length of K=20 samples (less than max restorable hole length=40)
-   M=25 intertwined blocks leading to 15 block sequences along the whole 30 seconds of ECG
-   a packet length of 256 bytes (according to the UWB link).

With such a coding scheme, simulation results showed that even for **8%** of packet losses the combined decoding/restoration scheme supported reconstruction of a more functional signal for a medical expert. In Figure 2, the first signal is the one including burst packet losses demonstrating the effect without interleaving coding (signal not available = holes); the second shows the same amount of losses demonstrating the effect obtained with the interleaving scheme and the latter the reconstructed signal. A specific zoom on the original signal, reduced losses and the reconstructed part is also presented.

The efficiency of the proposed restoration scheme was proposed to medical experts who recognized the efficiency of the process if the reconstructed parts were specifically labelled.

3. Conclusions

The URSAFE project has allowed the development of signal processing algorithms at two levels. Firstly, ECG event detection algorithms have been implemented and tested. According to the medical review, particularly performed with the atrial fibrillation behaviour (often considered as the most difficult condition to analyse), the obtained results are really satisfying. Indeed the specific correlation between medical signal assessment and automated results is very high. Secondly, the URSAFE project has pointed out a very important feature of biomedical signal transmission. Since no end-to-end network exists, some losses and delay may occur in data transmission, resulting in 1- 2 % (GPRS) or 8% (Satellite) packet losses (because medical experts cannot wait indefinitely for the retransmission of lost packets). To address this problem, we have proposed an interleaving of sample blocks within packets before transmission in order to reduce the length of successive missing samples at the receiver. Then, restoration algorithms have been tested on ECG signals and have provided promising results.

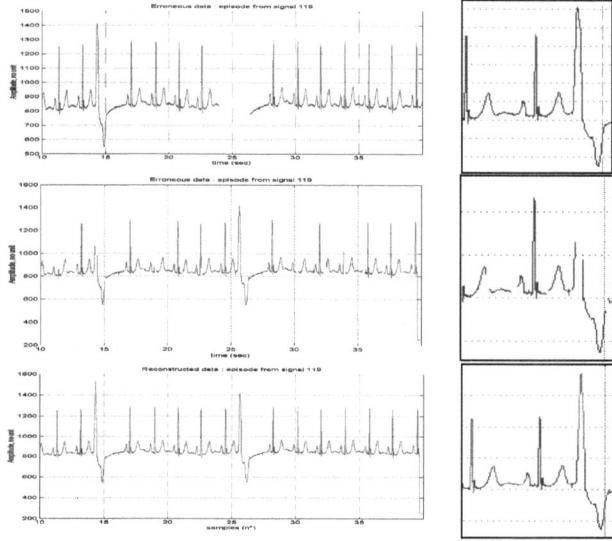

Figure 2 : Effect of interleaving and signal reconstruction.

References

[1]   B-U Köler, C. Hennig, R. Orglmeister, "The principles of software QRS detection", *IEEE Engineering in medicine and biology*, January/February 2002.

[2]   G. M. Friesen, T. C. Jannett, M.A. Jadallah, S.L. Yates, S. R. Quint, H. T. Nagle, "A comparison of the Noise sensitivity of Nine QRS detection Algorithms", *IEEE Trans BME*, vol. 37, n°1, January 1990.

[3]   J. Pan, W.J. Tompkins, "A real- time QRS detection algorithm", *IEEE Trans BME*, vol. 32, n°3, 1985.

[4]   M. Chabert, "Detection et estimation de ruptures noyées dans un bruit multiplicatif – approches classiques et temps echelles", *INPT PhD*, decembre 1997.

[5]   Marvasti, Nonuniform Sampling : theory and practice, *Kluwer Academic/Plenum Publishers*, NY, 2001.

[6]   P.J.S.G. Ferreira, Interpolation and the Discrete Papoulis-Gerchberg Algorithm, *IEEE Trans SP*, vol 42, n 10, October. 94, pp 2596-2606.

[7]   P.J.S.G. Ferreira, Interpolation in the time and frequency domains, *IEEE Signal Processing Letters*, vol 3, n 6, June 96, pp 176-178.

Personalised Health Management Systems
C.D. Nugent et al. (Eds.)
IOS Press, 2005

IT-based Diagnostic Instrumentation Systems for Personalized Healthcare Services

Honggu CHUN, Jaemin KANG, Ki-jung KIM, Kwang Suk PARK, Hee Chan KIM
Dept. of Biomedical Engineering, College of Medicine and
Center for Advanced Biometric Research Center,
Seoul National University, Korea

Abstract. This paper describes recent research and development activities on the diagnostic instruments for personalized healthcare services in Seoul National University. Utilizing the state-of-the-art information technologies (IT), various diagnostic medical instruments have been integrated into a personal wearable device and a home telehealthcare system. We developed a wrist-worn integrated health monitoring device (WIHMD) which performs the measurements of non-invasive blood pressure (NIBP), pulse oximetry (SpO_2), electrocardiogram (ECG), respiration rate, heart rate, and body surface temperature and the detection of falls to determine the onset of emergency situation. The WIHMD also analyzes the acquired bio-signals and transmits the resultant data to a healthcare service center through a commercial cellular phone. Two different kinds of IT-based blood glucometer have been developed using a cellular phone and PDA(personal digital assistant) as a main unit. A blood glucometer was also integrated within a wrist pressure measurement module which is interfaced with a cellular phone via Telecommunications Technology Association (TTA) standard in order to provide users with easiness in measuring and handling two important health parameters. Non-intrusive bio-signal measurement systems were developed for the ease of home use. One can measure his ECG on a bed while he is sleeping; measure his ECG, body temperature, bodyfat ratio and weight on a toilet seat; measure his ECG on a chair; and estimate the degree of activity by motion analysis using a camera. Another integrated diagnostic system for home telehealthcare services has been developed to include a 12 channels ECG, a pressure meter for NIBP, a blood glucometer, a bodyfat meter and a spirometer. It is an expert system to analyze the measured health data and based on the diagnostic result, the system provides an appropriate medical consultation. The measured data can be either stored on the system or transmitted to the central server through the internet. We have installed the developed systems on a model house for the performance evaluation and confirmed the possibility of the system as an effective tool for the personalized healthcare services.

Keywords. Telehealthcare, e-healthcare, personalized healthcare, diagnostic medical devices, Electrocardiongraph(ECG), blood glucose meter, blood pressure meter.

Introduction

A new concept of "personalized healthcare" or "personalized medicine" has emerged as a next generation medical service from the advancement and convergence of life science and information technology during the last decade. Even though the recent achievements in genomics, proteomics, molecular biology and bioinformatics are thought to unexpectedly change the shape of future diagnostics and therapeutics, many diagnostic medical devices integrated with increasingly smarter information technology (IT) are now being evaluated as a telemedicine or telehealthcare to provide more cost-effective, user-friendly and higher quality of medical services.

Research activities on telemedicine and telehealthcare in Korea have grown considerably from 1990s with advancement and expansion of the domestic IT infrastructure. As an example, telehealthcare center at the Seoul National University Hospital has been providing telemedicine services to the Seoul National University and 50 model houses using ISDN (Integrated Services Digital Network). Over 1,200 patients have examined and 83% of them replied that the service was satisfactory and 93% replied that the service was easy to use. In spite of this partial success in model telehealthcare services, there remain many technical, societal, and legal problems to be solved before we fully enjoy the advantages of this new medical service system. Standardizing the medical information, protecting the privacy of patients, establishing a guideline for proper level of medical charge, and clarifying the legal obligation are among the issues still unresolved. In technical view point, we need to develop standardized methods to interconnect the existing and forthcoming medical devices and various kinds of IT devices.

There have been a lot of research activities related to integrate various medical instruments with IT devices for telemedicine and/or telehealthcare services in the Department of Biomedical Engineering and the Advanced Biometric Research Center, Seoul National University. Main focus has been concentrated on the development of new IT-based diagnostic instrumentation systems in order to provide easiness in use for the possible users. Two different types of wearable systems and stand-alone systems have been developed for mobile and home use, respectively. Wearable systems include a wrist-worn integrated health monitoring device (WIHMD), three different types of IT-based glucometers. Non-intrusive health monitoring devices and a multi-functional integrated diagnostic system have been also developed and installed in a model house. All developed devices and systems were evaluated their performance to provide real-time automatic diagnosis and medical consultation not only to the patients with chronic disease such as cardiac disease, respiratory disease, diabetes and hypertension but also to the healthy but health-concerned subjects.

1. Materials & Methods

1.1. Wrist-worn Integrated Health Monitoring System for Telemedicine and
Telehealthcare

It is recognized that promptness of treatment is the most critical factor in emergency situations. Recent studies have shown that early and specialized prehospital management contributes to emergency case survival. The prehospital phase of management is of critical importance [1]. When an emergency occurs to an old person who lives alone, it's probable that he/she may have fallen and may remain for a long time without any treatment. Therefore, a real-time monitoring system with a tele-reporting function is required and we developed a WIHMD [Figure 1][2]. This system detects the fall and measures blood pressure, ECG, heart rate, respiration rate, body surface temperature and SpO$_2$. The WIHMD detects the fall of a patient by analyzing signals from a 2-axis accelerometer and an in-house fabricated posture sensor that is composed of a photo-interrupter with a pendulum. NIBP is measured by an oscillometric method based on the pressure signal from a wrist-cuff. Single channel ECG (LEAD I) is measured using textile electrodes which are located on inside and outside of the wrist-cuff for contacts with left and right hand, respectively. Heart rate and respiration are obtained by analyzing the ECG signal. Body surface temperature is measured by a semiconductor temperature sensor which is attached inside of the wrist-cuff. SpO$_2$ is measured using a finger-clip-type sensor which is connected to the main system. The WIHMD is linked to a cellular phone using an RF module (433MHz) and transmits the measured data to a healthcare center through the cellular phone using a Short Message Service (SMS). We have applied the system to ten volunteers for performance evaluation and confirmed the possibility of the system as an effective tool for telemedicine. Test methods and result are shown in Table 1.

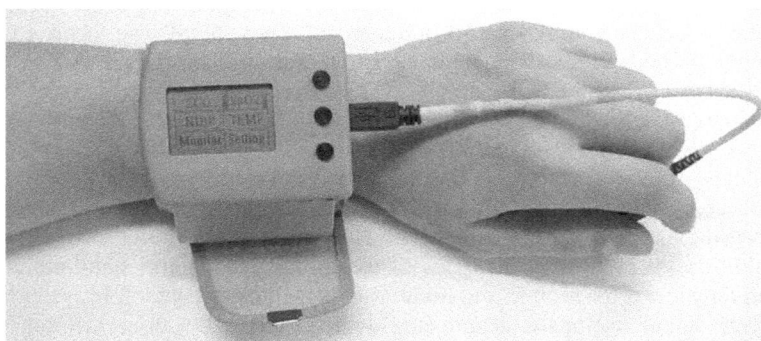

Figure 1. A wrist-worn integrated health monitoring device (WIHMD). This system detects fall and measures blood pressure, ECG, heart rate, respiration, body surface temperature and SpO$_2$.

Table 1. Summary of performance evaluation results of the WIHMD.

	Evaluation method	Number of tests	Test results
NIBP	Simulator (BPPump2M, Bio_tek, USA)	100	Error within ±4mmHg
SpO$_2$	Simulator (Oxitest plus7, DNI Nevada Inc, USA)	100	Error within ±2%
Heart rate from ECG	Simulator (PS214B, DNI Nevada Inc, USA)	100	Mean error 0.9%
Respiration from ECG	Human trial (WebDoc Spiro™, Elbio Inc, Korea)	50	Mean error 1.8%

Body surface temperature	Test set-up (Temperature-controlled chamber)	20	Mean error 1.5%
Falling	Human trial	150	Detection rate 91.3%

1.2. IT-based Blood Glucometers

Frequent measurement of blood glucose level is the most important diagnostic procedure for the diabetic patients. Even though the existing glucometers are portable with storage of a certain amount of measurement data, they do not provide fully satisfactory performance for mobile applications. A new glucometer connected to modern telecommunication devices such as a cellular phone and a PDA phone can remarkably enhance the user interface as well as the measured data management capabilities and can be carried at any time and any place. Once the blood glucose level is stored in such a telecommunicating device, the data can be easily transmitted to a remote server in healthcare service center through the possible combination of CDMA network, wireless LAN, and internet for further processing and services.

As shown in Figure 2, we have developed three different types of IT-based glucometers. In a PDA phone based system, the glucose measurement module was integrated into the PDA's main circuitry internally. For a cellular phone, we developed an external blood glucose measurement module that is interfaced via TTA standard. Therefore, this module can fit any kind of cellular phone produced in Korea. One can measure his/her blood glucose level and blood pressure easily in the third type device where a glucometer is integrated with a wrist-type blood pressure meter. This device also interfaces to a cellular phone via the TTA standard. By using a cellular phone or a PDA phone as a user interface, a larger display and more convenient functions can be achievable. A schematic diagram of the healthcare service model using those IT-based glucometers is shown in Figure 3. Measured data can be transmitted to a healthcare center, which consult with the patient using SMS. This type of service will be fully opened in Korea in April 2005.

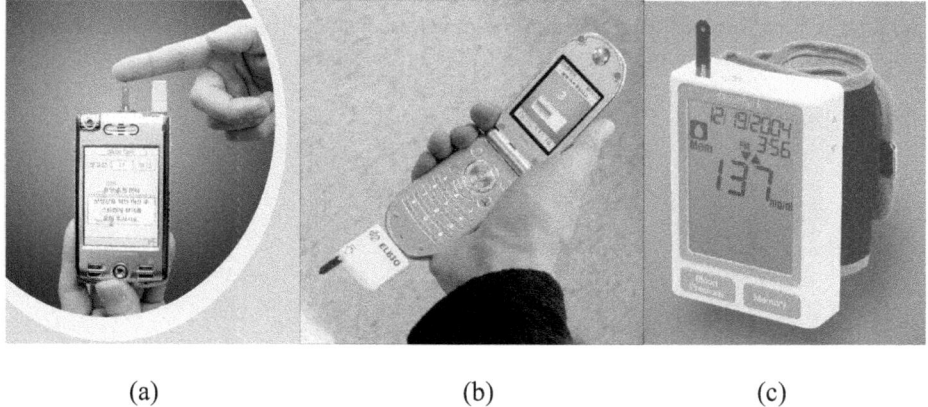

(a)   (b)   (c)

Figure 2. Three different types of IT-based glucometers; (a) PDA phone with an internal blood glucose measurement module, (b) an external blood glucose measurement module using TTA standard, and (c) a wrist-worn module for the measurements of blood glucose level and blood pressure.

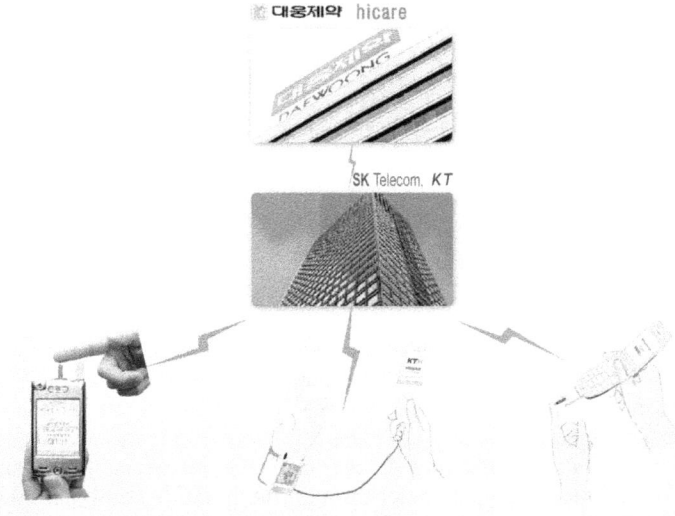

Figure 3. A healthcare service model using a cellular phone. One can measure his/her blood glucose level and/or blood pressure easily with one of the developed IT-based glucometers and then get an medical consultation through short message service (SMS) from the healthcare service center.

1.3. C. Non-intrusive Measurement of Biological Signals

Most of the existing medical instruments need the intention of a user to measure bio-signals and it is usually difficult to use correctly without a medical personnel's assistance. This may restrict the wide application of the personalized healthcare service system. A possible solution to this problem is non-intrusive measurement, which means the measurement of bio-signals without disturbing patient's ordinary activities, without cooperation for the measurement, and without patient's awareness of the measurement. The method can use any device we have to contact in a daily life for the measurement of bio-signals, which includes a bed, a toilet seat, a bath tub, shoes, a watch, a chair, a car seat, a belt, clothes and so on. We developed such non-intrusive measurement systems and installed them in a model house [Figure 4].

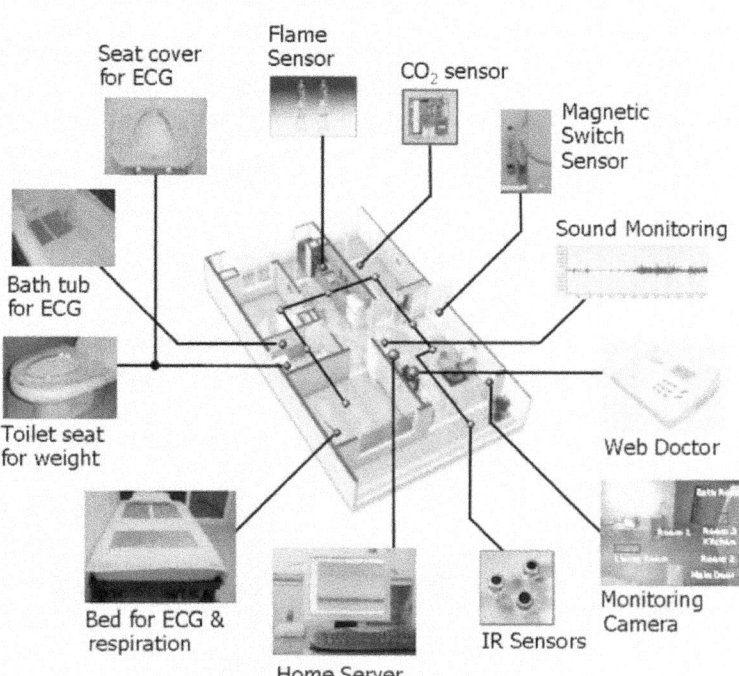

Figure 4. Model house for non-intrusive measurement of bio-signals. One can measure   ECG on a bed while he is sleeping; ECG, body temperature, bodyfat ratio and weight on   a toilet seat; ECG on a chair; the degree of activity by motion analysis using a camera.

Figure 5 shows a non-intrusive ECG measurement on a bed. The bedcover is made of three electrodes using copper coated conductive polyester textile. The user does not need to attach electrodes on his body to measure the ECG signal without any discomfort. We also successfully extract the respiration signal from the measured ECG waveform.

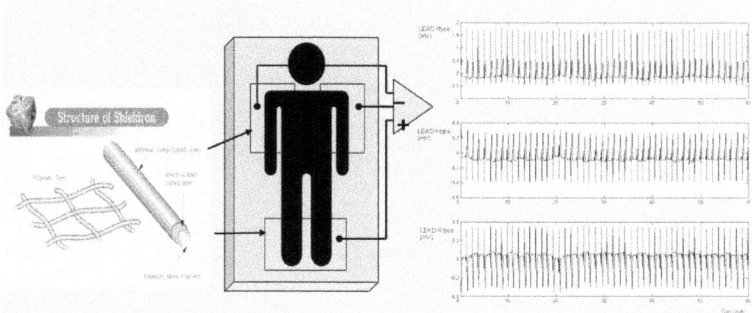

Figure 5. Non-intrusive ECG measurement on a bed using copper coated conductive polyester textile. Respiration signal is obtained by analyzing the ECG signal.

Figure 6 shows parameters that can be possibly obtained using a special toilet seat for non-intrusive measurement. Among those parameters, we developed a system that can measure the heart rate, body weight, body fat, body surface temperature and SpO_2. When a user sits on the toilet seat, it measures the body weight using imbedded load cells,   body surface temperature using a temperature sensor, ECG and pulse rate using copper coated conductive polyester textile, and SpO_2 using reflective type oxymetry sensor. All of these measurements are processed non-intrusively and automatically.

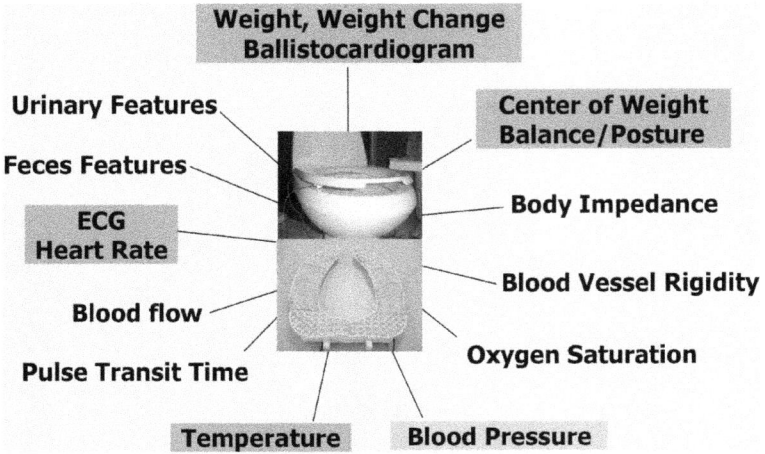

Figure 6. Parameters that can be possibly obtained from a specialized toilet seat. We developed a system that can measure the heart rate, body weight, body fat ratio, body surface temperature and SpO_2.

Copper coated conductive polyester textile was used as a useful material for non-intrusive bio-potential measurement. However, as conventional bio-potential measurement methods, it still requires a good contact between the electrode material and patient's skin. Sometimes, we need to measure bio-potential signal without touching a target object. A possible solution to this situation is a non-contacting capacitive bio-potential measurement. It utilizes insulated conductive plates as sensor to detect the changes in bio-potential [Figure 7]. We developed a non-contacting capacitive ECG measurement system on a chair [Figure 8]. A user can measure his/her ECG during working hours even in normally dressed condition.

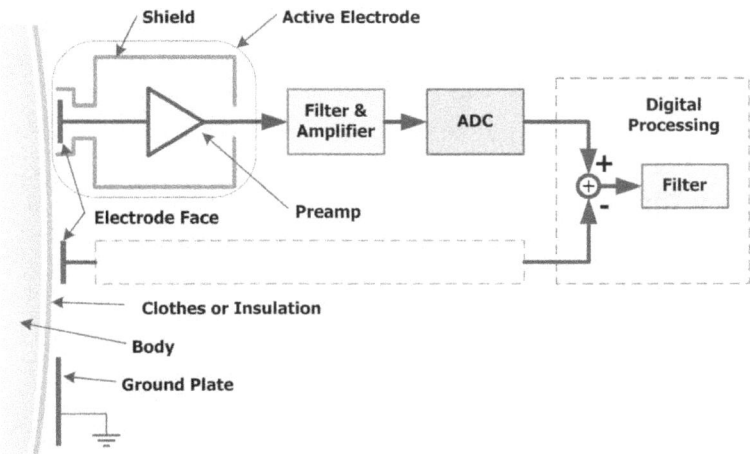

Figure 7. Conceptual diagram of non-contacting capacitive bio-potential measurement. It utilizes insulated conductive plates as sensors to detect the changes in bio-potential.

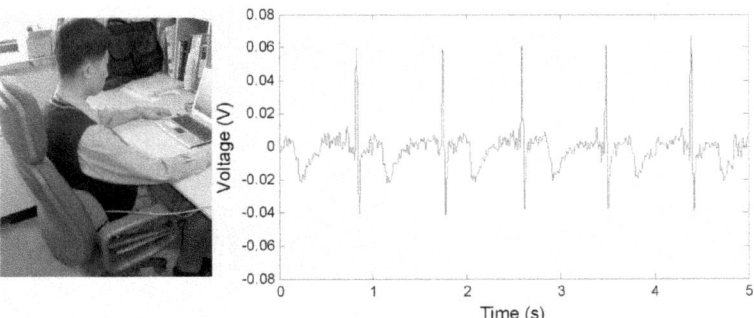

Figure 8. Developed system for non-contacting capacitive ECG measurement. It is installed on the back of a chair.

1.4. Development of an Integrated Home Telehealthcare System

In all the previously described systems, the main function of the developed device is to acquire user's health parameters and to transmit them to the central server in a healthcare service center through the telecommunication network. Then, the central server analyzes the data and diagnoses the current state of the patient, and then provides an appropriate teleconsultation or medical service if it is required. An integrated health monitoring system which not only measure the health parameters but also generate diagnosis and appropriate medical consultation can be useful for home telehealthcare services. This type of system would be especially beneficial to the people living in an area with poor infrastructure of telecommunication network. For this purpose, we have developed an expert health monitoring system for telehealthcare service to be used as a stand-alone system at home without any connection to a central healthcare server. This system is equipped with real-time automatic diagnosis and consultation function for patients with chronic disease such as cardiac disease, respiratory disease, diabetes and hypertension [Figure 9]. The system measures the standard 12-channel ECG, respiratory function, blood glucose level, and NIBP. The measured data are either stored on the system or transmitted to the central server if it is connected through the Internet. If there is any abnormality in the diagnostic result, the system generates a real-time alarm and an appropriate teleconsultation or medical service as well as sends a notice with measured data to the healthcare center.

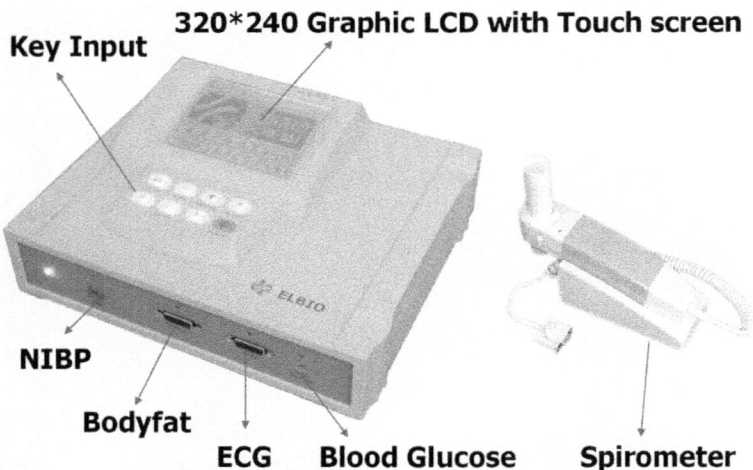

Figure 9. An integrated home telehealthcare system equipped with real-time automatic diagnosis and consultation functions. It measures standard 12ch ECG, respiratory function, blood glucose level and NIBP.

The system offers a convenient guide for the measurement by providing graphical instruction at every stage on a 320*240 graphic LCD with touch screen. Measured data are analyzed in real time and the diagnostic results are shown on the LCD with appropriate medical consultation. ECG measurement is required for the analysis of cardiac function of patient with chronic heart disease. ECG measurement module of the system was designed to meet the safety specification of IEC 60601-1, IEC 60601-2-25 and performance specification of KS P 1202-7. It acquires standard 12-channel ECG data for 10 sec and estimates parameters such as heart rate, PR interval, QRS duration, QT/QTc and P-R-T axes. Then it executes automatic diagnosis for heart abnormality over 200 cases related to rhythm, hypertrophy, QRS axis, conduction abnormality, myocardial infarction and ST-T abnormality. Spirometry is required for the analysis of respiratory function of patients with chronic respiratory disease. Spirometry module was designed to meet the safety specification of IEC601-1 and performance specification of KS P 1222. It can examine FVC(forced vital capacity), SVC(slow vital capacity) and MVV(maximum voluntary ventilation) with specified respiration protocol. At every measurement it estimates about 20 parameters related to volume and flow. Then it provides diagnostic results of the respiratory function of patient. Continued measurement of blood glucose level is required for patient with diabetes. Blood glucose meter module of the system was designed to meet the safety specification of IEC601-1 and the measurement error to be within 6.5%. It uses 0.5 µ l of capillary blood collected from a finger. Measured blood glucose level is shown with the history data in a chart form. The system diagnoses the current state of patient considering patient ' s history on diabetes and postprandial time. Continued measurement of NIBP is required for patient with hypertension. NIBP measuring module of the system was designed to meet the safety specification of IEC601-1 and performance specification of EN1060, KS P 6012 and IEC 601-2-30. And it meets the specification of SP10 recommended by Association for the Advancement of Medical Instrumentation (AAMI). Patient can measure one's blood pressure by wrapping the cuff on left upper arm. The system measures systolic pressure, diastolic pressure and heart rate. Measured blood pressure is shown with the history data in a chart form. The system diagnoses the current state of patient considering patient's history on blood pressure. The measured data can be either stored on the system or transmitted to the central server with the diagnostic result through the internet. The data size of transmission was 96 kbyte per full measurement of ECG, spirometry, blood glucose level and NIBP.

The developed system was installed in a model house and connected to the central server through the Internet. The central server was located at the Advanced Biometric Research Center (ABRC) of Seoul National University Hospital which was 1 km apart from the apartment. Whenever any resident member used one of the measuring modules, the original waveform with diagnostic results are stored on the system and transmitted to the central server everyday. Then, a medical expert at the healthcare service center reviews the transmitted data and offers teleconsultation if required.

2. Conclusion

We have developed the IT-based diagnostic instrumentation systems for personalized healthcare services. Utilizing the state-of-the-art information technologies, various diagnostic medical instruments have been integrated into a personal wearable device and a home telehealthcare system. The WIHMD which measures NIBP, SpO_2, ECG, respiration rate, heart rate, and body surface temperature and the detection of falls can be used for emergency detection for the high-risk patients or old-age people in mobile applications. Three different types of IT-based glucometers were developed to assist the diabetic patients and healthy people to easily measure and effectively manage their blood glucose level together with blood pressure. Another integrated diagnostic system for home telehealthcare services has been developed to include a 12 channels ECG, a pressure meter for NIBP, a blood glucometer, a body fat meter and a spirometer. An expert system measures health parameters and generate real-time diagnoses and appropriate medical consultation.

We have installed the developed systems on a model house for the performance evaluation and confirmed the possibility of the system as an effective tool for the personalized healthcare services. Patients who have used this system showed the response that they felt the sense of security with the real time diagnostic result and medical consultation function of the system. We expect this system will contribute to the realization of the personalized healthcare as a future medical service system.

Acknowledgment

This work is in part the result of research activities of Advanced Biometric Research Center (ABRC) supported by KOSEF.

References

[1]   B. Meade, "Emergency care in a remote area using interactive video technology: a study in prehospital telemedicine", Journal of Telemedicine and Telecare, vol. 8, pp.115-117, 2002.

[2]   J. Kang, J. Park, D. Park and H. Kim, "Development of a wrist-worn integrated health monitoring device for emergency telemedicine", 1st international symposium on e-health care, 2002, pp.5-8

[3]   Jeong RA, Hwang JY, Joo S, Chung TD, Park S, Kang SK, Lee WY, Kim HC, "In vivo calibration of the subcutaneous amperometric glucose sensors using a non-enzyme electrode", Biosens Bioelectron, 2003 Dec 15;19(4):313-9.

Personalised Health Management Systems
C.D. Nugent et al. (Eds.)
IOS Press, 2005

Networking and Data Management for Health Care Monitoring of Mobile Patients

Giuseppe AMATO [a], Stefano CHESSA [a b], Fabrizio CONFORTI [c],
Alberto MACERATA [c d, 1], Carlo MARCHESI [c e]

[a] *Istituto di Scienza e Tecnologie dell'Informazione, CNR, Italy*
[b] *Dipartimento di Informatica, Universita' di Pisa*
[c] *Istituto di Fisiologia Clinica, CNR*
[d] *Dipartimento di Medicina Interna, Universita' di Pisa*
[e] *Dipartimento di Sistemi e Informatica, Universita' di Firenze*

Abstract. The problem of medical devices and data integration in health care is discussed and a proposal for remote monitoring of patients based on recent developments in networking and data management is presented. In particular the paper discusses the benefits of the integration of personal medical devices into a Medical Information System and how wireless sensor networks and open protocols could be employed as building blocks of a patient monitoring system.

Keywords. Wireless Sensor Network, Health Care, Medical Device, Interoperability.

Introduction

ICT has been employed in medicine and health care for many years now with great success. However, the upgrade of existing medical instruments and the design of new medical applications as a result of continuous advances in information technology must not lead to neglect the real needs of patients and physicians. In this respect, ICT has failed so far to fully respond to requirements related to *integration* and *approach methodologies*. Although significant progress has been made in design and realisation of new medical instruments, the possibility of integrating these instruments with arbitrary operational information systems to build a single framework of healthcare resource is far to be realised.

Nowadays, personal medical devices (PMD) such as spirometers, glucometers, sphygmomanometers, pulse-oximeters and electrocardiographs are widely available on the market for self-monitoring purposes. However, in most cases, they are stand-alone products not integrated into a general framework of a Medical Information System (MIS). It should be observed that integration is particularly critical in order to be able

---

[1] Corresponding Author: Alberto Macerata, Istituto di Fisiologia Clinica CNR, via Moruzzi 1, 56100 Pisa (Italy); E-mail: macerata@ifc.cnr.it

to provide efficient medical support. In fact, different medical devices and hospital databases using different protocols and/or data representations may be unable to interact automatically and cannot be effectively used together.

The integration of PMDs in the MIS will allow a personalization of PMDs (exploiting patient information available from the MIS databases), the production of new patient medical data (obtained by combination of different PMDs), and an automatic enrichment of the MIS Electronic Patient Record.

The integration of data, as obtained by different PDMs, and their combination with environmental information could provide new information about the patient history which would not be available from a single PDM alone and constitutes reference data identifying the patient's patho-physiological behaviour in specific activity patterns.

A new scheme for cooperation between data, devices and systems is needed to be able to exploit simultaneously different patient related components, like PMDs, environmental data, GPs and hospital clinical data, financial and health care resources data. Although the current technologies offer the necessary means to singularly manage all these components, in our opinion it should be possible to access and integrate all the available health care resources offering a continuous, widespread, cooperative health care system and tools for personalized patient monitoring.

To achieve this, the current view of a medical instrument as a stand-alone device needs to be rethought; it should become a node in a medical network providing results and acquiring external data in order to update its internal knowledge in order to provide customized signal/data processing and patient-oriented answers.

In this paper we discuss the benefits of such integration and how it can be achieved. We will also highlight how the use of open protocols is fundamental for a successful integration.

The rest of the paper is organized as follows. Section 1 presents an example of an application scenario, Section 2 shows how wireless sensor networks can provide support to medical applications, Section 3 describes a network architecture to support such application scenarios and Section 4 will show how this architecture can support advanced signal processing. Perspectives in the design of a Wireless Sensor Network (WSN) based monitoring system are drawn in Section 5.

1. A Reference Scenario

Let us consider the scenario of a patient being remotely monitored at his home after hospitalisation for cardiac infarction. The patient's cardiac activity (i.e. the heart rate and peripheral blood pressure), body temperature and breathing frequency should be continuously monitored. In addition, alert situations should be automatically detected and notifications should be sent to proper destinations (for instance an expert physician) in order to take immediate actions. However, all this monitoring activity should be hidden and transparent to the patient: he/she should be guaranteed a good quality of life.

This hidden remote monitoring is not easily obtained. Consider that the health condition of a patient can only be partially evaluated through his vital signs and must be mediated and integrated by other information coming both from personal characteristics (risk factors, degree of disease, age, sex, family history, psychological profile, etc.) and from the environmental context (i.e. whether in bed or mobile, by him/herself or in company, at work or at home, the season and the temperature, etc.).

The monitoring system should be able to provide feedback to the patient as well as notifying his status to somebody else, such as a relative, the family doctor, or the hospital, depending on the degree of alert detected, and possibly adapting the level of service (i.e. the intensity of the monitoring activity).

2. Wireless Sensor Networks

2.1. State of the Art and Research Directions in Wireless Sensor Networks

We believe that effective remote monitoring of patients can be obtained through the exploitation of WSN technology. A WSN [1] is composed of a set of low cost, low power microsystems (sensors) equipped with sensing devices and a wireless network interface. The recent proliferation of research on WSNs has been motivated by the need for flexible and efficient environmental monitoring. Typical existing applications of sensor networks are environment sampling, monitoring disaster areas, surveillance, security, inventory management, and they have also been envisioned as a means of architectural support for applications of pervasive computing. We believe that WSNs can also be satisfactorily used for patient monitoring. A platform for sensor network based on MICA2® technology is presented in [2].

The sensors of a WSN collect information about the surrounding environment (*sensor field*) and provide sensed data to external *sink nodes*. To this purpose the sensors can be programmed according to different paradigms which define the communication model between the sensors and between the sensor network and the sinks. In the most known paradigm (called *data diffusion*) [3] the network is organized into a directed acyclic graph rooted in the sink, and the sensed data flow with different rates from the sensors to the sink. However, in the effort of improving the management of the streams of data produced by sensor networks, it has recently been proposed to integrate database and sensor network technologies [4].

This integration however offers a new vision of the sensor networks and of the database technologies. On the database side, it should be considered that data streams produced by the sensors hardly adapt to the data model of a traditional database. One important difference is that a traditional database deals with a set of data that can be considered static as compared to data that needs to be managed in a sensor network. Even if a database is able to deal with evolving data sets, the evolution rate of data produced in a sensor network is much higher than that typically managed by database systems. Besides, in traditional databases data are stored in a persistent repository and can be accessed at any time. Query languages, query optimisation strategies, and query processing strategies are based on this assumption. On the other hand, given the limited amount of memory and the energy constraints of the sensors, data should be processed in real time and acquired just when needed. Data streams produced by the sensors might be processed by (smart) sensors themselves, but in this respect the strategies of query optimisation and query processing should also be redefined. Finally query languages should reflect this new way of handling data.

Furthermore, the state of the art architectures of sensor networks are quite unfeasible to support databases. Given the constraints of the sensor device, the design of a system oriented to sensor networks and database technologies for data processing should proceed alongside.

2.2. A Sensor Network Architecture Supporting Advanced Data Management

Based on the MICA2® technology, we developed a network and middleware prototype layer for sensor networks, which support the execution of queries produced by the sink nodes; work on a prototype of database is in progress.

In our model, the sink issues queries (written in a declarative language such as an SQL extension), which are optimised and distributed over the sensor network. These queries specify monitoring, data collection and/or processing tasks with different levels of intensity. They also define the flux of information between sensors. The queries are translated into query execution plans expressed in terms of an extended relational algebra. The translation and optimisation of queries are performed by the sink node from where the query originates. The final query execution plan divides the original query into sub-queries and defines the allocation of sub-queries on the sensors, with the aim of choosing the lowest execution cost.

Each sensor is thus assigned a sub-query defining the set of sensors providing the data streams necessary to execute the sub-query and the rules to combine such streams. At this level, communication between sensors is implicit since sensors only use operations to open, read or write local or remote data streams. At a lower level, opening a remote data stream implies that the data produced on a remote sensor should be routed and buffered at the local sensor.

The sensors manage streams via the middleware layer (called the *stream system*), which provides support for the management of local and remote data streams and for stream buffering and naming, and exploits the services of the network layer for routing.

The network layer provides support to the communication models used by the stream system (unicast and multicast). It defines a *virtual coordinate system* [5] which assigns a coordinate to each sensor in the network and allows efficient geographical routing. The virtual coordinate system is hop-based and unrelated to the physical location of the sensors. Thus it does not require sophisticated equipment to find coordinates and has little overhead. The network layer also embeds an *energy efficiency management* [6] module, which turns off the wireless interface during periods of inactivity. These periods are computed taking into account the requirements of the network and the stream system layers.

3. Network Architecture

3.1. Multilevel Medical Network

Monitoring of patients is needed in different environmental situations: in a clinical infrastructure, at home, while jogging or travelling. This requires a flexible network infrastructure that allows sensing units to communicate with the available network facilities.

The MIS, managing the PMDs, has to be organized into layers with the patient at the centre (Figure 1). The inner layer which provides monitoring support could be viewed as a Body-Area WSN. This network, hosted by the patient, combines the patient's physiological data with information from the outer layers to support (basic) early diagnosis and to produce (basic) alerts. The outer layer (for example the patient's domotic or vehicular local network) may include an environmental sensor device and/or one or more powerful nodes such as PDAs, PCs or external diagnostic devices, able to collect data, to manage advanced monitoring and alert the detection service. This new layer interacts with the outermost layer (i.e. HIS) to exchange physiological data, alerts and patient related data (Figure 2). Wireless connections should be used where possible to support mobility and adaptability at the various levels of the network.

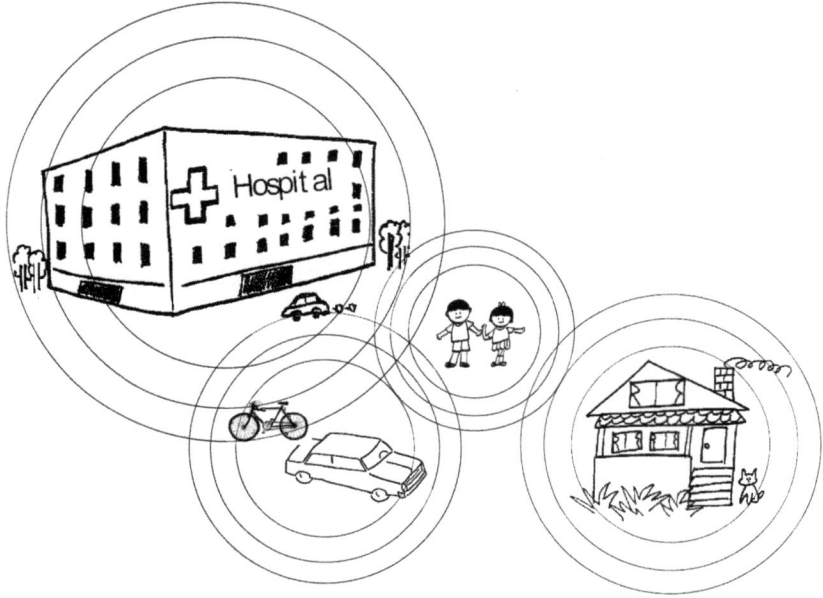

Figure 1. Wireless Sensors Network coverage and data integration.

3.2. Open Protocols for Data Exchange

Nowadays, PMDs use none or, at best, different and proprietary standards for data transfer or exchange. No automatic integration of data among different types of PMDs exits, at least in devices among different manufactures. Integration is typically performed by medical personnel through visual inspection of output data.

Network integration of PMDs with a reference data collector, like HIS database, could offer a continuous and detailed history of patients so covering the gap in between different accesses to the hospital. This can be a promising improvement toward the solution of the challenging problem of the Patient Medical Record.

Open communication protocols in PMDs management and data exchange is mandatory[7-9]. The availability of an open protocol will promote its use in commercial devices and support interoperability in hospital, at home and in enlarged social/health care services.

In this open context the standards that are already available and commonly used in medical devices and communications should be adopted; liaisons with international standard development organizations should be pursued especially with the eHealth Focus Groups (HL7, IHE, DICOM, OpenECG).

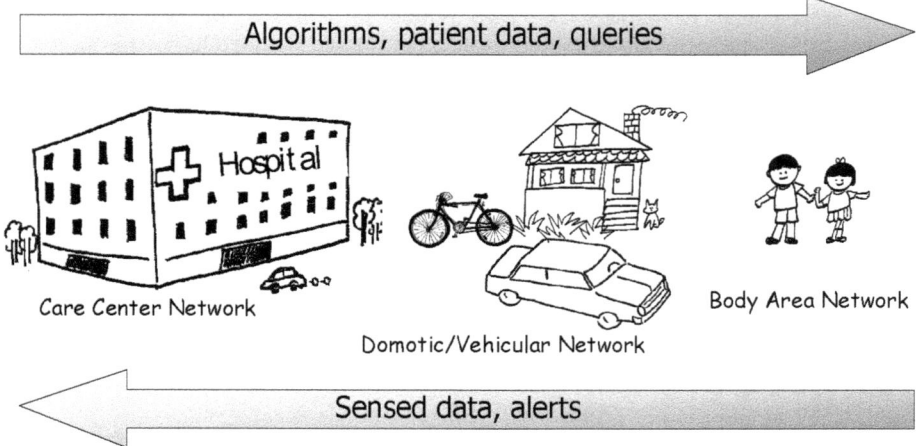

Figure 2. Flow of WSN data through different network layers.

4. WSN Cooperative Signal Processing

Computing and storage capabilities, as offered by sensor network nodes, are limited but not irrelevant. In fact, basic signal processing such as synchronization, filtering and compression can be implemented at the sensor level.

Other more complex tasks, such as signal feature extraction, data fusion or decision support, should be performed through the co-operative work among nodes and exchanging pre-processed data so the workload among sensors is balanced. In case of limited resources for computing or input/output facilities a PDA can be added to the network for extra processing power and, for instance, as interface for displaying warning messages to the patient and manual input of data.

Moreover, the outside patient network layers (domotic and HIS networks) could offer information for extracting new cross-parameters and combinatory feature arrays which could improve the reliability of patient feedback, local warnings and alarms.

5. Virtual Personal Medical Device

The design of a new sensor based monitoring system requires the knowledge of the users' requirements (patients and healthcare operators) and of data processing specifications taking into account the technical constraints like data flow, communication speed and frequency band, network protocols, computation requirements, time delays and battery capacity.

Moreover, this system has to be adapted to different kinds of patients with different pathologies and disease severities, different conditions of life and activities, living in different environments and with the availability of different technical infrastructures or network coverage. All these conditions require different types of sensors, different data processing, specific alarms and different support or data interchange with other nodes or external worlds with different communication requirements.

If the WSN infrastructure seems to be able to manage all the technical aspects for patient monitoring it will be able to support advanced signal processing by gaining from the patient profile and history as stored in a reference HIS database.

The flexibility of this kind of architecture should allow the composition of different modules into a new virtual PMD according to the patient monitoring requirements and hardware/network resources.

References

[1] I.F. Akyyildiz, W. Su, Y. Sankarasubramaniam, E. Cayirci: Wireless sensor networks: a survey, Computer Networks 38 (2002), 393–422.

[2] Crossbow Technology, "MICA wireless measurement system datasheet", www.xbow.com/Products/Product_pdf_files/Wireless_pdf/MICA.pdf

[3] C. Intanagonwiwat, R. Govindan, D. Estrin: Directed diffusion: a scalable and robust communication paradigm for sensor networks, Proceedings of the ACM Mobicom, Boston, MA (2000), 56–67.

[4] S. Madden, M.J. Franklin, J.M. Hellerstein and W. Hong: The Design of an Acquisitional Query Processor For Sensor Networks, Proceedings of the ACM SIGMOD, San Diego, CA (2003), 491–502.

[5] A. Caruso, S. Chessa, S. De, and A. Urpi: GPS Free Coordinate Assignment and Routing in Wireless Sensor Networks, Proceedings of the IEEE INFOCOM, Miami, FL (2005).

[6] G. Amato, P. Baronti, S. Chessa: Application-Driven Energy Efficient Communication Model in Sensor Networks, in preparation.

[7] http://www.gnu.org/home.html

[8] http://www.italy.fsfeurope.org/documents/freesoftware.en.html

[9] http://softwarelibero.it/documentazione/softwarelibero.shtml

V. Community Health 2

Personalised Health Management Systems
C.D. Nugent et al. (Eds.)
IOS Press, 2005

Lifestyle Support Through Efficient ECG Acquisition and Analysis

Steven DEVLIN, Chris NUGENT, Dewar FINLAY
School of Computing and Mathematics, Faculty of Engineering
University of Ulster at Jordanstown, Northern Ireland, BT37 0QB

Abstract. People are becoming more aware of their health and the lifestyles they live. As people use computers more and more in a wide variety of occupations, they would find it desirable to monitor their lifestyle without having to leave their desk. Through the analysis of the Electrocardiogram (ECG), it is possible to obtain a person's heartrate and diagnose a number of conditions associated with abnormal heart function [1]. To obtain an accurate heartrate, the ECG signals have to be analysed and calculations performed to find occurrences of the QRS complex, a major component of the ECG signal. This research entailed creating the software required to interpret ECG signals recorded from an innovative computer peripheral allowing recordings from the user's forearms as they operate the computer. The user could therefore effortlessly monitor their lifestyle during normal computer usage.

Keywords. Lifestyle System, Lifestyle Monitoring, Electrocardiogram Analysis.

Introduction

A larger percentage of the population than ever before are making the effort to pursue a healthier lifestyle by eating healthier food, doing more exercise and monitoring their lifestyle. Lifestyle is defined simply as how one lives [2] and a lifestyle system can be thought of something that helps one monitor how they live. This paper reports the development of a non-invasive lifestyle system to allow individuals to monitor health related parameters during normal and regular computer usage.

An advanced innovative computer peripheral that allows ECG signals to be recorded from the user's forearms as they operate the computer is in development. The aim of this research was to develop an application to execute in the background of the variations of the Microsoft Windows Operating Systems, while providing the user regular feedback of their heartrate. The application would also provide a method of viewing this information graphically and retrieving a history of recorded data that can be viewed on a daily, weekly or even monthly basis to assess lifestyle trends.

1. Lifestyle Monitor Application

A computer peripheral currently in development allows ECG signals to be recorded from the user as they operate a computer. This is possible through the use of a specially adapted keyboard which records the user's ECG signals from their forearms through electrodes that are incorporated in the wrist support area of the keyboard. The ECG signals that are recorded from these electrodes on the keyboard are transmitted to the computer, following analogue to digital conversion, using the RS232 Serial Port.

1.1 Lifestyle Monitor Application

The purpose of the Lifestyle Monitor application is to process the ECG signals received from the keyboard and provide the user with regular notifications of their heartrate. This process involves transforming the received signal into practical information for the user, allowing them to not only view instantaneous notifications of their heartrate, but also to examine a more in depth graphical representation of the obtained information on a daily, weekly or monthly basis.

1.2 User Environment

For an application to succeed in the mainstream consumer market, a necessary feature is that it is compatible with the Microsoft Windows environment. This is based on the fact that all variations of the Microsoft Windows Operating System account for 93.8%[1] of the consumer desktop operating system market worldwide.

Early in the development stages of the Lifestyle Monitor, the benefits of focusing on one Operating System family as opposed to providing support for multiple platforms was considered. It was concluded that by doing so, it was possible to have a much closer integration with the Operating System, which in turn provided scope for improved functionality and enhanced features.

All development was undertaken using the Microsoft Visual Studio .NET 2003 development environment.

1.3 ECG Acquisition & Analysis

The application interacts with the computer's RS232 Serial Port to obtain the user's raw ECG signal. In order to obtain the subject's heartrate and further subsequent diagnostic information, a series of processing steps are conducted. The first step is to locate the occurrence of one cardiac cycle, i.e. a heartbeat, which allows the identification of a reference point in the ECG waveform. The 'R' peak of the 'QRS' complex should be the most prominent feature of an ECG waveform in terms of amplitude [3], and this point was used as a reference in this application. By identifying the peak of the R wave in successive cycles the R-R interval [4], as illustrated in Figure 1, can easily be measured which in turn allows the calculation of the heartrate.

---

[1] Based on the online magazine, INTERNETWEEK.com, column published in 08th October 2003 'Windows Gains Market Share, Despite Linux Threat', that highlights the market share of various operating systems in 2002.

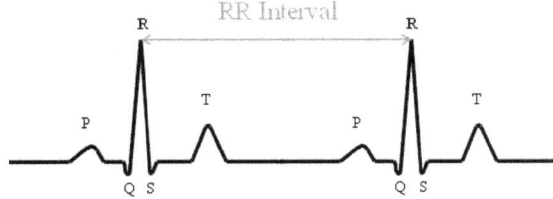

Figure 1. The ECG, Highlighting a R-R Interval.

1.4 Background Execution

The application is designed to operate in the background whilst the user is conducting normal tasks. In order to provide seamless integration with the windows environment, the user interface of the application was incorporated in the Windows system tray. This is the area at the bottom right of the Windows Graphical User Interface (GUI), to the left of the Clock. The Lifestyle Monitor Icon is circled in Figure 2.

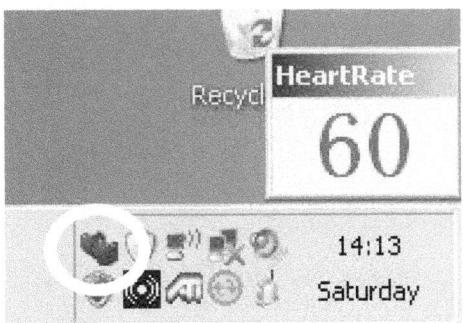

Figure 2. Lifestyle Monitor Executing in the Background of Normal
Windows Usage, Heart Rate Notification displaying at 100% Opacity.

While executing in the background, the application provides notifications to the user of their current heartrate. Figure 2 is a screenshot of the notification displayed to the user. The notification is designed to appear above the Windows System Tray as a pop-up message. To ensure this can always be seen, the application checks the user's current screen resolution and location of the Start Bar and sets the coordinates of the notification accordingly. The notification display interval and duration can be defined by the user, as can the opacity of the pop-up window. This allows the user to have greater control over the notification functionality. The opacity option allows the user to have a more subtle notification, right down to 30% opacity allowing the heartrate to be visible while still being able to observe the window beneath the notification.

1.5 Main Interface

The main interface of the application allows the user to graphically view their recorded data. It is possible to view the current day's heartrate, as well as the raw data which is currently being recorded from the computer peripheral. A screen shot of the graphical displays can be seen in Figure 3. The application also keeps a 'heartrate' history of each individual that uses the computer. Each day the application records information for a user. At a later date the user is then able to select a date and view the recorded data graphically for that day. This can be seen in Figure 4.

The main interface is accessible from the execution icon displayed in the Windows System Tray. The user can set their individual preferences from either the System Tray icon or from the main interface.

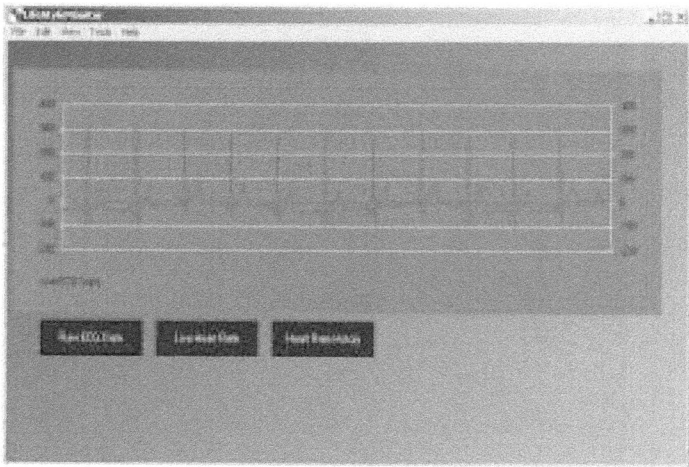

Figure 3. Raw ECG Data Graphical Display.

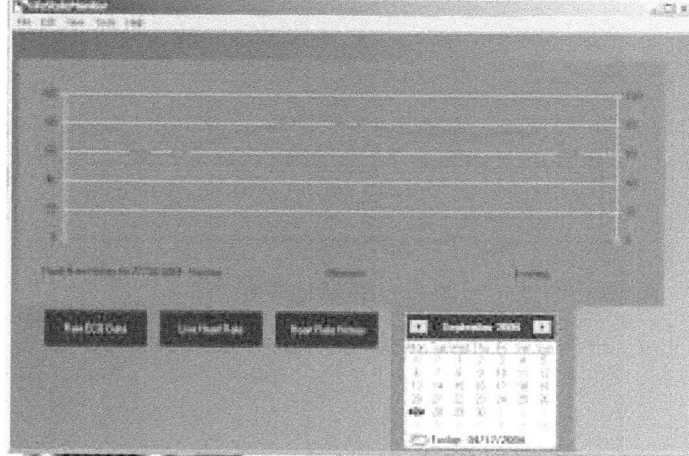

Figure 4. Heartrate History & Date Picker.

1.6 Integration with Windows Registry

The application is designed to work closely with the Windows Registry, and this relationship provides much of the functionality of the application. Firstly, the application is capable of operating without the need for a main user interface. From the application executing in the System Tray, the user automatically receives heartrate notifications. The application also retrieves information about the current screen resolution and location of the start bar to find the display location of the notification. The user can 'Right-Click' the System Tray icon to access a menu that allows tasks to be executed, again without accessing the main interface. This is shown in Figure 5.

Another aspect that exploits the Windows Registry is the support of multiple users of the application. Each user's settings, including pointers to heartrate history data, are stored in the Windows Registry, under the 'Current User' tree. This means that each user account on the computer has its own settings for the Lifestyle Monitor application.

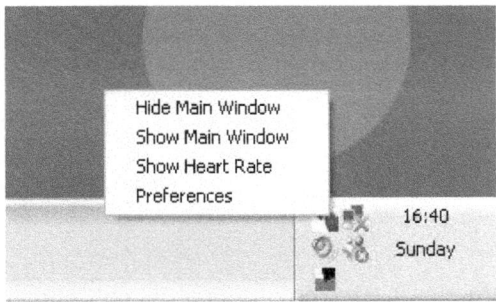

Figure 5. Menu Accessible from
'Right-Clicking' the System Tray icon.

2. Conclusion

By introducing the Internet to this project, the possibility of integration with existing e-Health solutions can be envisaged. .The application could be developed to allow for remote observation of patients who may be at risk of heart disease. This could be achieved through the implementation of a Web Service to collate information from a patient's application and allow this information to be graphically available to the patient's doctor or clinician. A conceptual view of this framework is shown in Figure 6.

The application developed allows lifestyle conscious people to further monitor and analyse their heartrate, without the need of physically wearing or consciously applying a device. It also provides scope for extension to a remote monitoring system, allowing patients to be observed from home or from their office by the clinician or doctor. The application's close relationship with the Windows Operating System allows for seamless execution, providing the user with unobtrusive regular notifications of their heartrate.

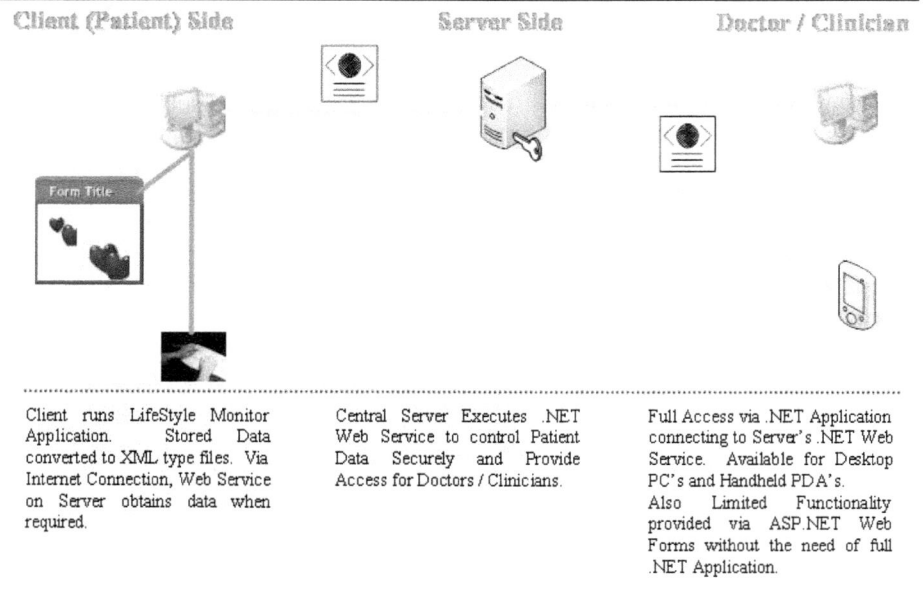

Client (Patient) Side	Server Side	Doctor / Clinician
Client runs LifeStyle Monitor Application. Stored Data converted to XML type files. Via Internet Connection, Web Service on Server obtains data when required.	Central Server Executes .NET Web Service to control Patient Data Securely and Provide Access for Doctors / Clinicians.	Full Access via .NET Application connecting to Server's .NET Web Service. Available for Desktop PC's and Handheld PDA's. Also Limited Functionality provided via ASP.NET Web Forms without the need of full .NET Application.

Figure 6. Lifestyle Monitor – Future Development Framework.

References

[1] Köhler, B.U. *et al*; The Principles of Software QRS Detection; IEEE Engineering in Medicine and Biology – Jan/Feb 2002 (Vol. 21, No. 1).

[2] http://www.cob.sjsu.edu/escudier_b/Spring%202003/MKT%20134A%20SP03/HAWKINS/Chapter %2012%20 Excersize %20and%20Questions.doc

[3] CD Nugent, JAC Webb, GTH Wright, ND Black, Electrocardiogram 1: Pre-processing Prior to Classification, Automedica, vol. 16, pp. 263-282, 1998.

[4] Hampton, J.R.; The ECG Made Easy; 4th Edition (1994); Churchill Livingstone; ISBN: 0-443-04507-0.

Personalised Health Management Systems
C.D. Nugent et al. (Eds.)
IOS Press, 2005

Non-Mediated Glucose Biosensing using Nanostructured TiO$_2$

Julie RANKIN, Tony BYRNE, and Eric McADAMS
Northern Ireland Bio-engineering Centre, University of Ulster, Newtownabbey,
Co. Antrim, Northern Ireland, BT37 0QB

Abstract. Insufficient insulin production in diabetics can be controlled by discontinuous measurement and insulin therapy. Ideally, an artificial pancreas system would be a closed loop system measuring glucose levels, and administering insulin as required, to minimise patient contribution. This paper presents an investigation into the use of titanium dioxide as an electrochemical transducer for the detection of hydrogen peroxide. Hydrogen peroxide is the product of glucose oxidation by the enzyme glucose oxidase in the presence of oxygen. The results show that peroxide can be quantitatively detected by electrochemical reduction on titanium dioxide electrodes without interference due to dissolved oxygen. When tested for the indirect amperometric measurement of glucose (with free glucose oxidase) it was found that the electrodes responded linearly over the range of glucose concentration found in human blood. With further development, these electrodes may be suitable for implantable glucose sensors.

Keywords. titanium dioxide, hydrogen peroxide, glucose oxidase, biosensor.

Introduction

Diabetes mellitus is a worldwide health problem, involving an insulin deficiency, which results in an inability to control blood glucose levels. About 2% of population (greater for over 40's) suffer from insulin deficiency. Type 1 diabetics cannot produce any insulin and are therefore dependent on insulin injections. Type 2 diabetics are able to produce limited amounts of insulin and therefore may not be dependent on insulin injections. Both types of diabetes involve the personal discontinuous measurement of blood glucose levels. This includes the use of lancets and finger pricking devices to take a sample of blood for determination of glucose in a sensing device. In more chronic cases of diabetes, insulin therapy usually involves a discontinuous administration of insulin 2-4 times a day by injection. Untreated diabetics are susceptible to long-term damage to the eyes, kidneys, nerves, heart and major arteries.

An ideal system would function as an artificial pancreas, utilising an implanted glucose sensor for the continuous on-line determination of blood glucose levels with feedback control of an insulin delivery system. This would reduce the requirement for patient involvement in both glucose monitoring and insulin injection, significantly, and would be an improvement in personal health care for diabetics.

Commercially available glucose sensors are biosensors. Biosensors are comprised of a biological detection element, a transducer, and a signal processor. The biological element should be selective to a specific substrate or group of substrates and enzymes are commonly used e.g. glucose oxidase (GOD) which oxidises glucose using oxygen as the electron acceptor. The reduction of oxygen results in the production of hydrogen peroxide (H_2O_2), which can be detected electrochemically either by oxidation or reduction. Most commercially available glucose biosensors involve the use of mediators for "electrical wiring" of the GOD enzyme to the electrode transducer. Briefly, the glucose is oxidised by GOD which itself becomes reduced (takes up electrons). The GOD_{Red} normally passes these electrons on to dissolved oxygen as the electron acceptor to form H_2O_2. However, in a mediated biosensor, one utilises a molecule or ion with a reversible redox couple i.e. the GOD_{Red} form passes the electrons on to the mediator which itself becomes reduced. The reduced form of the mediator can then be oxidised (electrons removed) at a suitable electrode. This oxidation of the reduced mediator is measured as an electric current that is therefore proportional to the glucose concentration. However, mediated glucose biosensors may not be suitable for *in-vivo* glucose sensing as the mediators used may be toxic, or simply lost by dissolution and diffusion into the blood. It is therefore desirable to look at the possibility of non-mediated glucose biosensing e.g using materials which can either be directly wired to the enzyme or which are selective for peroxide, the product of glucose oxidation in the presence of oxygen.

If H_2O_2 can be detected in the presence of oxygen, without interference, there is an opportunity to produce a wide range of biosensors, utilising oxidase enzymes. Figure 1 shows a schematic representation of how an electrochemical biosensor for glucose might operate. The use of mesoporous titanium dioxide electrodes has been reported previously for the amperometric detection of glucose via electro-reduction of released hydrogen peroxide [1].

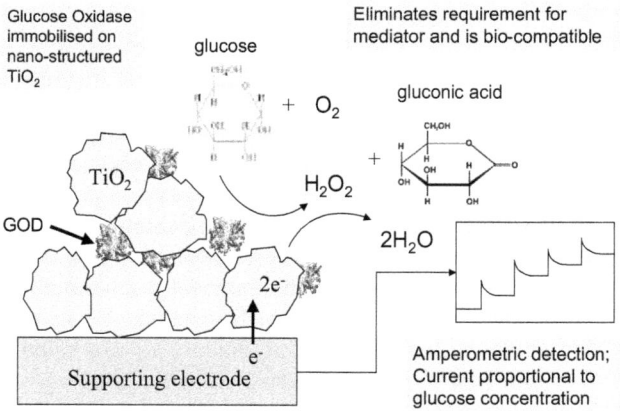

Figure 1. Schematic diagram of operation of non-mediated electrochemical biosensor.

The photocatalysis group at University of Ulster has developed an electrophoretic coating procedure to give porous nanocrystalline TiO_2 electrodes [2,3]. These electrodes have been tested for the electrochemical reduction of H_2O_2 in the presence of O$_2$ and the response is independent of O$_2$ at potentials more positive than –0.4 V versus saturated calomel electrode (SCE).

1. Experimental Details

1.1. Reagents

Titanium dioxide (Degussa), HPLC grade Methanol – (Riedel de Haen), 30 % hydrogen peroxide solution (BDH), Phosphate buffer made from monobasic sodium phosphate (BDH) and dibasic sodium phosphate (BDH). Glucose oxidase (from *Aspergillus niger*, Sigma).

1.2. Methods

Titanium foil samples were cleaned by sonication in hot detergent solution followed by several rinses in distilled water. The samples were coated with nanoparticle TiO$_2$ by the electrophoretic method previously reported [3]. Electrical contact was made to an area of the Ti foil which was not coated with TiO$_2$ using a copper wire and conducting epoxy. The contact and any remaining uncoated foil area were insulated using a negative photoresist.

All electrochemical analysis was carried out using a three-electrode electrochemical cell, with pH 6 phosphate buffer as the supporting electrolyte. The reference electrode was saturated calomel (SCE), and the counter electrode was a platinum disc. Dissolved oxygen concentration was controlled either by air sparging or oxygen free nitrogen (OFN) sparging of the buffer solution. Cyclic voltammetry experiments were performed using an Autolab PGSTAT20 potentiostat/galvanostat. The fixed potential current measurements were carried out using a BAS LC-4C amperometric detector connected to a Lloyd instruments PL3 x-y plotter. All potentials are reported against SCE at room temperature and atmospheric pressure.

2. Results and Discussion

2.1. Linear Sweep Voltammetry (LSV)

As glucose is oxidised by glucose oxidase, H$_2$O$_2$ is produced. The biosensor must be able to detect the reduction of the H$_2$O$_2$ by-product without interference due to the reduction of O$_2$. Initial studies investigated the reduction of H$_2$O$_2$ on the TiO$_2$ electrodes. Figure 2 shows the electrode response determined using LSV in the presence and absence of O$_2$ and/or H$_2$O$_2$.

The reduction current in the presence of H$_2$O$_2$ (Figure2 (c)) was greater than that observed in the presence of O$_2$ alone (Figure 2 (b)). The onset potential for H$_2$O$_2$ reduction was less negative than that for the onset of O$_2$ reduction. However, in the presence of both H$_2$O$_2$ and O$_2$, the reduction current was greater than that for H$_2$O$_2$ alone. In LSV the current observed is a mixture of both capacitive and faradaic components. In order to separate these components one can measure the current time response at a fixed potential.

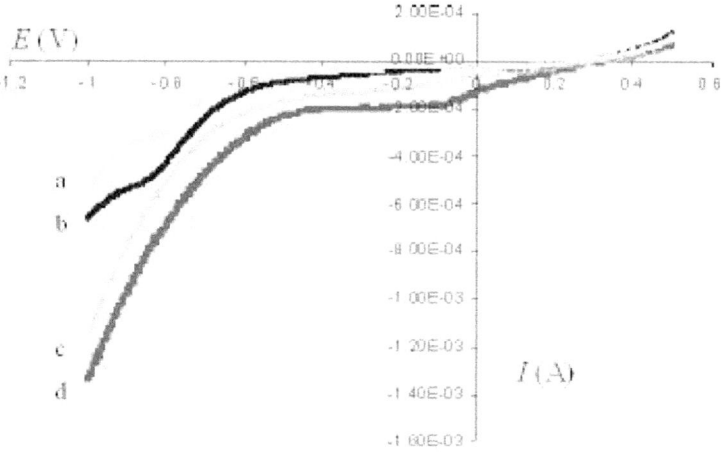

Figure 2. LSV of TiO₂ electrode in pH 6 phosphate buffer. The potential was swept from +0.5 V to –1.0 V at 20 mV s⁻¹. (a) buffer, (b) O₂ only, (c) H₂O₂ only, (d) H₂O₂ and O₂. O₂ concentration was ca. 11 mM and H₂O₂ concentration was 0.0012 M.

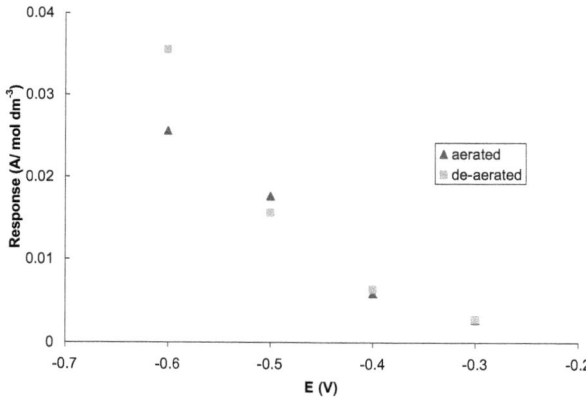

Figure 3. Measured amperometric response of TiO₂ electrode in pH 6 phosphate buffer to H₂O₂. Applied E constant for each experiment. O₂ concentration was controlled by either air sparging or OFN sparging of the buffer solution.

2.2. Amperometric Detection at Fixed Potential

The electrode response due to H₂O₂ in the presence and absence of O₂ was determined using amperometry at fixed potentials over a range of potentials i.e. -0.3 V, -0.4 V, -0.5 V and –0.6 V. Figure 3 shows the steady state current as a function of electrode potential. At potentials more negative than – 0.4V, the cathodic current was greater in the air sparged solution than in the OFN sparged solution. However, at –0.4 V there was no difference in the current response to H_2O_2 either in air sparged or OFN sparged solution. Therefore, H_2O_2 reduction can be determined on a TiO_2 electrode at a fixed potential of −0.4 V with negligible interference from O_2 reduction.

2.3. Response to Glucose

Glucose oxidase was added to the buffer (air sparged) in free suspension, and the electrode response was measured at −0.4 V. Standard additions from a stock solution of glucose were made to the cell and the steady state current measured. The steady state current as a function of glucose concentration is shown in Figure 4. The glucose oxidase oxidises the additions of glucose to produce H_2O_2, which is then reduced at the TiO_2 electrode. The electrode response was directly proportional to the glucose concentration over the 2 mM to 20 mM glucose.

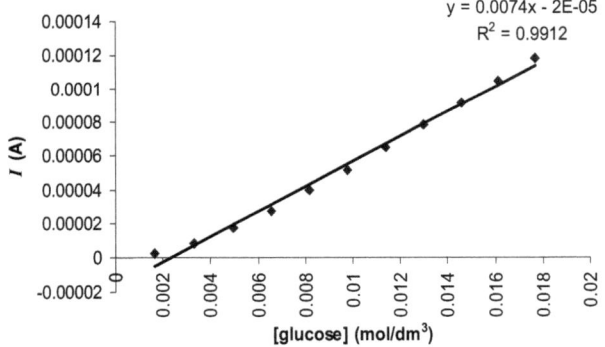

Figure 4. Electrode response to standard additions of glucose. 10 mg GOD was present as free enzyme in 30 cm³ pH 6 phosphate buffer. The TiO_2 electrode was held at a fixed potential of -0.4 V.

3. Conclusions

The concentration of glucose found in physiological blood is in the range of 2 mM to 25 mM. Therefore, a sensor for glucose must respond over that concentration range and more preferable give a linear response. Nanostructured TiO_2 electrodes may be used as electrochemical transducers for the detection of H_2O_2 in the presence of O_2 without interference from O_2 reduction at an applied potential of −0.4 V. Also, the current response of the electrode was directly proportional to glucose concentration when glucose oxidase enzyme was present as free enzyme in the buffer solution.

As TiO_2 is biocompatible these electrodes, incorporating immobilised glucose oxidase, may be suitable for use as implantable glucose sensors. Furthermore, TiO_2 electrodes could be used as electrochemical transducers for a wide range of biosensors utilising oxidase enzymes. Work is ongoing investigating different routes to the immobilisation of glucose oxidase onto the surface of nanostructured TiO_2.

Acknowledgements

The Department of Employment and Learning for funding J. Rankin's research. Degussa for supplying samples of P25.

References

[1]   S Cosnier, C Gondran, A Senillou, M Gratzel, N Vlachopoulos, "Mesoporous TiO$_2$ Films: New Catalytic Electrode Materials for Fabricating Amperometric Biosensors Based on Oxidases", *Electroanalysis*, 1997, **9(18)**, 1387-1392.
[2]   J A Byrne, B R Eggins, S Linquette-Mailley and P S M Dunlop, "The effect of hole acceptors on the photocurrent response of particulate titanium dioxide", *Analyst*, 1998, **123**, 2007-2012.
[3]   J A Byrne, B R Eggins, N M D Brown, B McKinney, and M Rouse, "Immobilisation of titanium dioxide for the treatment of polluted water", *Applied Catalysis B: Environmental*, 1998, **17**, 25 – 36.

Personalised Health Management Systems
C.D. Nugent et al. (Eds.)
IOS Press, 2005

Detection and Removal of Pathogenic Biofilms on Medical Implant Surfaces

Patrick DUNLOP[1], Louise OLIVER, Tony BYRNE, and Eric McADAMS
Northern Ireland Bio-Engineering Centre, University of Ulster at Jordanstown, U.K.

Abstract. Advances in sensor technology have had a significant impact in medical research and practice in the last decade. However, within the hospital environment problems still exist where the application of sensing technology could provide the solution. The presence of antibiotic resistant bacteria within hospitals and the risk of serious infection that they pose is a cause for concern. This paper describes a research project that has recently started at the University of Ulster investigating the potential of "Sense and Destroy" tactics to reduce the spread of medical device related infections. It is proposed that Electrical Impedance Spectroscopy (EIS) probes implanted within a catheter may be used to detect sub-clinical biofilm formation. Furthermore, if the presence of a biofilm is detected, activation of a photocatalytic coating on the catheter wall may be used to inactivate the responsible microorganisms.

Keywords. Electrochemical Impedance Spectroscopy, photocatalysis, MRSA, Hospital-acquired infection.

Introduction

Advances in sensor technology have had a significant impact on the fields of medical and biomedical research and medical practice in the last decade. Clinicians are now dependent upon these technologies to aid in diagnosis, monitor patient's vital signs, and reduce time taken for bodily fluid analysis. Bedside monitoring is now commonplace and developments in diagnostic instrumentation allow the patient to monitor their condition, and take appropriate action, from the comfort of their own home.

Within the hospital environment problems still exist where the application of sensing technology could provide the solution. The presence of antibiotic resistant bacteria within hospitals and the seriousness of the infection that they can cause, are a growing concern. Hospital-acquired infections (HAI) are defined as infections that are neither present nor incubating when a patient enters hospital. Their effects vary from discomfort to prolonged or permanent disability and they may contribute directly or substantially to a patient's death [1]. A recent report by the World Health Organisation found an average of 8.7% of hospital patients developed nosocomial infections during

---

[1] Corresponding Author: PSM Dunlop, Northern Ireland Bio-engineering Centre, University of Ulster, Shore Road, Newtownabbey, Co. Antrim, Northern Ireland. BT37 0QB Email:psm.dunlop@ulster.ac.uk

their time in hospital [2]. It has been estimated that HAI costs the NHS in England £1 billion per year. Not all HAI are preventable but Infection Control Teams believe that they could be reduced by at least 15%, with yearly savings of £150 million [3]. Hospital acquired bacteraemia and line-sepsis, accounting for just below 10% of all HAI, are undoubtedly associated with significant mortality. Almost two thirds of bacteraemias are associated with an intravascular device, with central intravascular catheters found to be the most common source. Catheters can become infected by a number of different routes with the infection proliferating in multiple areas along the catheter surface.

A recent study reported that over 40% of the identified microorganisms causing hospital-acquired bacteraemia were Staphylococci, with over half of the *Staphylococcus aureus* isolated being resistant to methicillin (ie. were MRSA) [4]. Pathogenic biofilms are extremely difficult to treat, often requiring the removal of the device and necessitate the use of reserved second or third line anti-microbial agents, which may not penetrate very well into the biofilm. Moreover the causative organisms of biofilm infections are frequently multiple-antibiotic resistant [5]. This paper describes a research study at the University of Ulster, in collaboration with the Royal College of Surgeons in Ireland, investigating the potential of "Sense and Destroy" tactics to reduce the spread of medical device related infections.

1. Project Aim

The aim of this research is to remove the risk of post-operative line sepsis and pathogenic bacterial biofilm recruitment on the surfaces of catheters and medical implants. The study involves two specific research projects:

1. *"Sense"- Using Electrical Impedance Spectroscopy (EIS) probes implanted within the catheter material for early detection of sub-clinical biofilm formation.*

EIS is a non-destructive electrochemical technique, commonly used to measure physical and chemical properties of a wide range of materials. This technique has previously been used to detect pathogens and is routinely used in sterility control in animal feed manufacture. EIS has also been used for microbial detection in aqueous environments, eg. bacterial contamination of milk and water. Research at the University of Ulster has shown EIS to be a suitable method for the detection of the initial stages of bacterial growth. Traditional microbial detection techniques require up to 24 hours to confirm bacterial presence however detection can be achieved in 4-6 hours using EIS (Figure 1). In this application EIS is used to identify the presence of pathogenic bacteria attaching to the electrode array imprinted on the catheter surface. Early detection of this attachment can allow hospital staff extra time to intervene before a biofilm is formed and the associated problems develop. In a clinical setting EIS electrodes on catheter tips are currently employed for the detection of heart valve and pumping volume problems [6]. Understanding the effects of miniaturisation of the EIS sensors is of critical importance in order to develop probes suitable for biofilms detection on catheter surfaces. To this effect a range of EIS probes have been designed and fabricated using bio-compatible materials (Figure 2). These are currently being analysed for their bio-impedametric properties and will ultimately be included in many positions within the catheter wall.

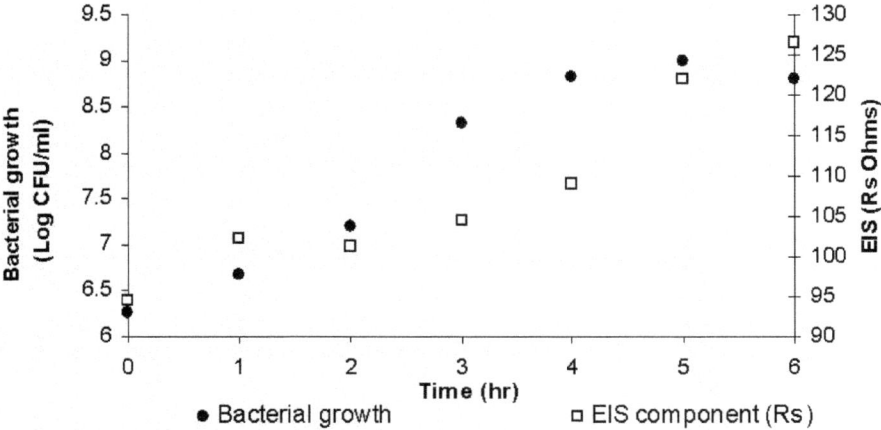

Figure 1 Bacterial detection using EIS. Value of EIS (Rs) increase with bacterial growth, significant changes in EIS (Rs) evident after four and five hours confirming bacterial growth at this early stage.

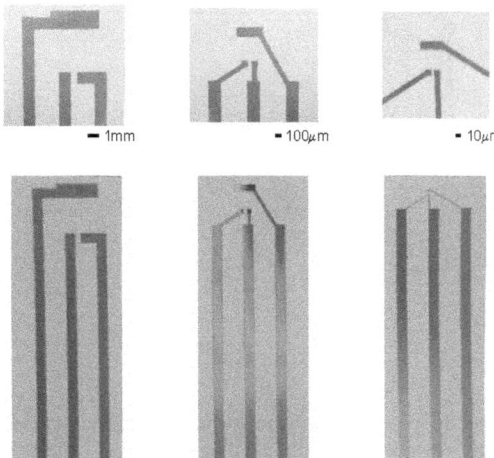

Figure 2 Miniaturised EIS probes designed to be incorporated into catheter walls. Photo: PSM Dunlop.

2.   "Destroy" - Coating catheters or medical implant surfaces with durable layers of photocatalytic materials and the activation of the coating.

Upon detection of an infection on the device clinicians can either treat the infection with antibiotics or replace the catheter.   Both of these methods increase patient discomfort, place an additional workload upon hospital staff, drain hospital resources and increase the patient's length of stay within the hospital.   Secondly, the infection may not respond to the antibiotics resulting in the eventual replacement of the device. An alternative may be to use photocatalytic coatings, which can inactivate bacteria when exposed to UVA irradiation.   Photocatalysis harnesses the power of a biologically inert catalyst, titanium dioxide (TiO$_2$), which upon irradiation with UV light can produce radical species capable of destroying microorganisms [7]. TiO$_2$ is a white powder commonly used as a pharmaceutical-bulking agent, in chewing gum and as a bleaching agent in a number of food products. The photocatalyst can be activated by UV light, however in the absence of irradiation TiO$_2$ returns to its biologically inert form. Photocatalysis has been shown to be effective against a wide range of gram positive and gram negative micro-organisms, including *Staphylococcus aureus,* which can develop into the super-bug MRSA [8]. When UV light strikes a semiconductor TiO$_2$ particle an electron is promoted from the valence band to the higher energy level conduction band, leaving behind a positively charged region called a "hole". The hole can react with water to produce hydroxyl radicals, very powerful oxidising species, which can inactivate bacteria. A schematic mechanism for photocatalytic disinfection is detailed in Figure 3.

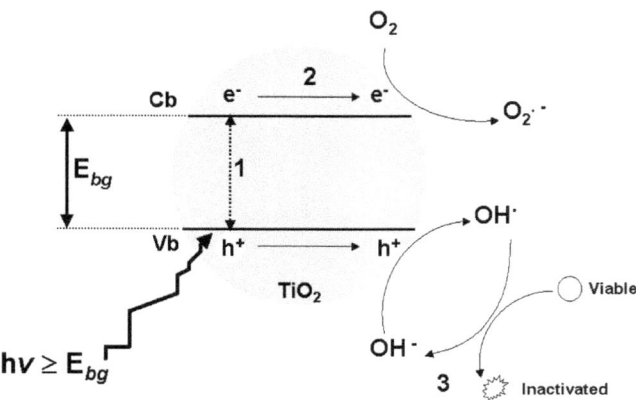

Figure 3 shows a schematic representation of photocatalytic disinfection.
1- Excitation of an electron (e⁻) from the Valence band (Vb) to the Conduction band (Cb) leaving positive hole (h⁺).
2- Migration of the charge carriers to the surface of the TiO$_2$ particle.
3- Production of hydroxyl radical (OH·) from water and subsequent inactivation of biofilm contamination.

Research is focused on the adaptation of photocatalysis to inactivate traditionally disinfectant resistant biofilms formed on the surface of the medical device. If the EIS sensors detect contamination, hospital staff can quickly introduce the UV source to activate the coating and destroy the causative agent and prevent serious infection. Consideration must be given to the effects of this treatment on internal features of the veins and the blood system, however given the nature of the surface specific radical generation in photocatalysis we expect that tissue damage will not be an issue.

2. Conclusion

The development of "smart" medical devices, which can sense and remove biofilm contamination, could play a significant role in the prevention of hospital-acquired infection. The project described in this paper is in its early stages of development, however benefits to patients, clinicians and the hospital managers are expected.

Acknowledgements

The authors would like to thank the HPSS R&D Office for funding this project in collaboration with the Royal College of Surgeons in Dublin under the Ireland – Northern Ireland Co-operation Project Grant scheme.

References

[1]   R.L. Smith, R.G. Sawyer, T.L. Pruett, Hospital-acquired infections in the surgical intensive care: Epidemiology and prevention, *Zentralblatt Fur Chirurgie*, **128** (2003), 1047-1061.

[2]   World Health Organisation (WHO). Prevention of hospital-acquired infections. A practical guide 2nd Edition, WHO/CDS/CSR/EPH/2002/12. Accessed 17/04/2003

       . http://www.who.int/csr/resources/publications/drugresist/WHO_CDS_CSR_EPH_2002_12/en/

[3]   R. Plowman, N. Graves, M. Griffin, The socio-economic burden of hospital-acquired infection. London: Public Health Laboratory Service 2000.

[4]   Anao, Surveillance of hospital-acquired bacteraemia in English Hospitals 1997-2001. London: Public Health Laboratory Service and Nosocomial Infection Surveillance Service 2001.

[5]   D.J. Diekema, M.A. Pfaller, F.J. Schmitz, J. Smayevsky, J. Bell, R.N. Jones, M. Beach, Survey of infections due to Staphylococcus species: Frequency of occurrence and antimicrobial susceptibility of isolates collected in the United States, Canada, Latin America, Europe, and the Western Pacific region for the SENTRY Antimicrobial Surveillance Program, 1997-1999, *Clinical Infectious Diseases*, **32** (2001), S114-S132.

[6]   W. Arthur, G.C. Kaye, Clinical use of intracardiac impedance: Current applications and future perspectives, *Pace-Pacing and Clinical Electrophysiology*, **24** (2001), 500-506.

[7]   A. Mills, S. LeHunte, An overview of semiconductor photocatalysis, *Journal of Photochemisty and Photobiology A-Chemistry*, **108** (1997), 1-35.

[8]   D.M. Blake, P.C. Maness, H. Zheng, E.J. Wolfrum, J. Huang, Application of the photocatalytic chemistry of titanium dioxide to disinfection and the killing of cancer cells. *Separation and Purification Methods*, **28** (1999), 1-50,

Personalised Health Management Systems
C.D. Nugent et al. (Eds.)
IOS Press, 2005

Development of a Virtual Reality System for the Rehabilitation of the Upper Limb After Stroke

Jacqueline CROSBIE[1], Suzanne McDONOUGH[1], Sheila LENNON[1]
and Michael McNEILL[2]

[1] *Health and Rehabilitation Sciences Research Institute, University of Ulster,*
Shore Road, Newtownabbey, Co. Antrim, BT37 0QB. NORTHERN IRELAND
[2] *Faculty of Engineering, University of Ulster,*
Cromore Road, Coleraine, Co. Londonderry, BT52 1SA. NORTHERN IRELAND

Abstract. Virtual reality (VR) provides a three-dimensional computer representation of a real world or imaginary space through which a person can navigate and interact with objects to carry out specific tasks. One novel application of VR technology is in rehabilitation following stroke, particularly of the upper limb. This paper describes the development of a VR system for use in this field. This system gives the user the ability to interact with objects by touching, grasping and moving their upper limb.

Keywords. Virtual reality assisted rehabilitation; stroke rehabilitation; upper limb; user perspectives.

Introduction

Virtual reality (VR) provides a three-dimensional computer representation of a real world or imaginary space through which a person can navigate and interact with objects to carry out specific tasks. It can be either *immersive*, where the user feels physically present in the virtual environment (VE), typically using a head-mounted display (HMD) or *non-immersive*, where a handheld interface allows interaction with objects on a computer screen. One novel application of VR technology is in rehabilitation following stroke, in this case of the upper limb. Recovery of upper limb function is a major problem, with 30 – 66 % of stroke survivors no longer able to use the affected arm [1]. This can be explained in part by the site of injury in the cortex [2], which can cause limb paresis that limits active practice with the arm in the real world [3]. Other factors are low levels of interaction between the patient and the environment [4, 5], ineffective therapy techniques [6], and the very small percentage of time actually spent practicing tasks [4]. After a stroke involving the upper limb, many patients naturally tend to use the more affected limb less, and the 'non-use' reinforces and contributes to the lack of use [7]. The facilitation of practice is very important as it has been reported in the rehabilitation literature that early [3, 8, 9] intensive [10, 11,

12] practice of active functional tasks [13, 14, 15] in an enriched environment [16, 17, 18, 19] leads to more positive outcomes for upper limb rehabilitation, by modifying neural reorganisation of the cerebral cortex [20, 21].

The use of VR technology has been advocated for this problem as it can be manipulated to avoid the physical constraints that would prevent a patient practicing in the real world and, also, the virtual environment can be tailored to suit individual movement problems and needs. In its immersive form visual, auditory and tactile sensory aspects of the VE can be delivered to the individual through visual display units and speakers within an HMD unit [22]. A tracking system can be used to link head movements so that the image in the VE is updated in synchrony with actual head movements, giving an impression of looking around from within the VE. In addition to this, a representation of the user's upper limb can be generated within the VE using sensors on the arm and a dataglove on the hand [23] so that the user can interact with objects as though they were real [24]. The aim of this study was to design and build a VR system for upper limb rehabilitation, which could be used by rehabilitation therapy staff i.e. non-professional computing personnel.

1. Equipment: Virtual Reality Rehabilitation System

Our research group has built a system for use in stroke rehabilitation, which gives the user the ability to move around a world composed of simple and familiar objects, and to interact with these objects by touching, grasping and moving their upper limb. The user wears a CyVisor HMD with built-in ear speakers, which supports visual and audio feedback and a 5DT data glove that facilitates manual interaction in the virtual world. An Ascension Flock-of-Birds magnetic sensor system provides real-time 6-degrees of freedom (position and orientation) tracking of up to four points on the user's body. A VE has been created with a series of reaching and grasping tasks. The user is seated in front of a table, which is replicated in the virtual environment and populated with a number of virtual markers and easily recognisable objects, for example cups and pencils (see Figure 1). The user sees a number of easily recognisable objects in addition to a stylised representation of their arm and hand in the VE, which replicates the movement of their upper limbs in the real world. Three sensors are attached to the major upper limb joints (shoulder, elbow and wrist) and the fourth is attached to the HMD to facilitate the sense of immersion in the VE. Functional tasks have been designed to incorporate a range of levels of difficulty for reach, grasp, release and manipulative components. The tasks engage both individual joint movements and the use of the whole arm and some require fine upper limb and hand motor control. They have been designed so that complex tasks can be divided into a number of smaller sub-tasks. A wrist extension task has been designed to focus particularly on the movement at this joint. It is likely to be functionally useful to promote wrist extensor activity as it impacts on grip strength and the dynamic positioning of the hand for grasping objects.

All patient movement is monitored and logged for post session analysis. All elements of the system and the users' interactions are measurable, so therefore the rehabilitation for each patient can be quantified over an extended period of use. The system set-up, configuration and user sessions can be performed by healthcare staff. After initial assessment the user participates in an introductory training session: The therapist takes the person through 'a guided tour' and shows them how the system works. Audible instructions and pre-recorded demonstrations can be played through the

HMD to briefly explain each task to the user. The user is then invited to try to move his or her arm to reach for a target object in the VE, for as long as they wish to practice. The user can practice a variety of tasks including reaching and grasping familiar shapes and objects such as a cup or glass.

Placement of all virtual objects is flexible and can be changed according to the individual's abilities to make the tasks easier or more challenging. The distance and height of the virtual objects can be altered in relation to the users' position. All arm and hand movements are tracked in real time and displayed to the user along with audio feedback to provide encouragement. Data is stored off-line for post session analysis. This can be used as video replay to show the user their performance and to allow them to check if any changes have been made in their movements.

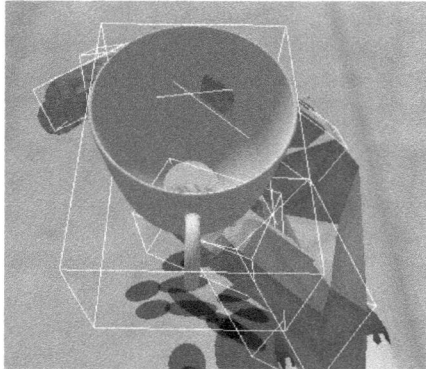

Figure 1: View of hand interaction with virtual cup.

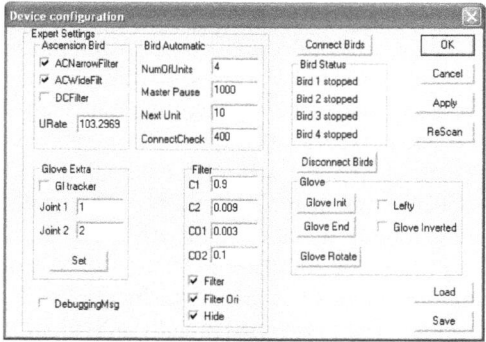

Figure 2: Dialogue box of system specifications.

With regard to the system configuration, the operator has access to a series of dialogue boxes, which enable the system specifications to be controlled and allows dynamic control of the testing and training situations (see Figure 2). Initially some user-specific data is loaded into the system e.g. length of arm, distance from elbow to hand etc. After assessment of the user's abilities, the positions of the virtual objects can be changed using the appropriate dialogue box or the keyboard. New positions can be stored along with the user-specific data in a session file. As a task is performed the operator monitors user progress and if necessary can adapt the structure of each task to suit the individual.

2. Pilot Testing of the System

The system is in the process of being tested on both healthy volunteers and users with stroke. The Queen's University Belfast Ethical Committee granted ethical approval. *Inclusion criteria* for those following stroke was: first stroke with a motor impairment of the upper limb as a primary deficit, muscle strength greater than 2/5 on the Medical Research Council (MRC) scale; stable medical condition; ability to communicate; good cognitive ability as indicated by a score greater than 15 on the Mini Mental State Examination (MMSE) [25], Motricity Index score [26] greater than 26 out of 100, indicating either activity of the shoulder or elbow and beginnings of prehension in the hand. Users with stroke who have significant dysphasia, severe hemiplegic arm pain, and severe visuo-spatial neglect on the Line Cancellation Test [27] are excluded. Informed written or witnessed verbal consent is obtained from all recruited patients and healthy adults.

Three outcome measures have been chosen. The Immersive Tendencies Questionnaire (ITQ) determines differences in the tendencies of individuals to experience presence [28]. A person with a positive immersive tendency might be more likely to be successful in the performance of virtual tasks. The Task Specific Feedback Questionnaire (TSFQ) questions the users' on their perception of the level of difficulty of the tasks carried out in the VE [29]. This instrument gives a total score of between 1 and 30. Lower scores indicate that the user had a more favourable experience in the VE. The Borg Scale of Perceived Exertion [30] was used to assess the individual's perception of any physical exertion they may have experienced whilst exercising their arm in the VE. A score of zero represents no perceived exertion or discomfort and 10 represents the greatest amount of perceived exertion that the person has ever experienced.

3. Conclusion

The VR system has been developed for rehabilitation of the upper limb in people after stroke over a 12-month period. The system has been tested to date on ten healthy adults and five people after stroke.f Preliminary analysis of data would seem to indicate that users in both groups had a generally favourable experience using the system, with equal numbers of users reporting either positive or negative immersive tendencies. The main difference between groups relates to the level of perceived exertion. The healthy group rated the experience of using the VR rehabilitation system as none to a weak level of exertion. Whilst the users with stroke perceived the level of exertion demanded to be at a higher level of moderate to strong.

Acknowledgements.

Northern Ireland Chest, Heart and Stroke Association, 6th Floor, 22 Great Victoria Street, Belfast BT2 7LX (Application number: 2002004).

References

[1]   J. H. van der Lee, R. C. Wagenaar and G. J. Lankhorst, Forced use of the upper extremity in chronic stroke patients, *Stroke,* **30** (1999), 2369-2375.

[2]   E.R. Kandel, J.H. Schwartz and T. M. Jessell, *Principles of neural science* (3rd edition), Prentice-Hall International Inc, London, 1991.

[3]   J. Chae, F. Berthoux and T. Bohine, Neuromuscular stimulation for upper extremity motor and functional recovery in acute hemiplegia, *Stroke* **29** (1998), 975-979.

[4]   D. J. Tinson , How stroke patients spend their days, *Int Disab Studies* **11** (1989),45-49.

[5]   F. Mackey, L. Ada and R. Heard, Stroke rehabilitation: are highly structured units more conducive to physical activity than less structures units? *Arch Phys Med Rehab* **77** (1996), 1066-1070.

[6]   G. H. Kraft, S. S. Fitts and M. C. Hammond, Techniques to improve function of the arm and hand in chronic hemiplegia, *Arch Phys Med Rehab* **73,** (1992), 220-227.

[7]   J Carr and R Shepherd, *Stroke rehabilitation. Guidelines for exercise and training to optimise motor skill.* Bitterworth Heineman, London, 2004.

[8]   D. T. Wade, V. A. Wood and R. Langton Hewer , Recovery after stroke – the first three months, *J of Neuroy, Neurosurg and Psych* **48** (1985),7-13.

[9]   B. B. Johansson, Brain plasticity and stroke rehabilitation, *Stroke* **31** (2000), 223-230.

[10]   P. Langhorne, R. Wagenaar and C. Partridge, Physiotherapy after stroke: more is better? *Phys Res Intern* **1** (1996), 75-88.

[11]   G. Kwakkel, R. C. Wagenaar, T. W. .Koelman, G. H. Lankhorst and J. C. Koetsier, Effects of intensity of rehabilitation after stroke: a research synthesis, *Stroke* **28** (1997), 1550-6.

[12]   G. Kwakkel, R. C. Wagenaar, J. W. R. Twisk, G. H. Lankhorst and J. C. Koetsier, Intensity of leg and arm training after primary middle-cerebral-artery stroke: a randomised trial, *Lancet (North American Edition)* **354** (1999), 191-6.

[13]   C. Dean and F. Mackey, Motor assessment scale scores as a measure of rehabilitation movement control following stroke, *Physio* **69** (1992), 238-240.

[14]   G. V. Smith, R. F. Macko, K. H. C. Silver and A. P. Goldberg, Treadmill aerobic exercise improves quadriceps strength in patients with chronic hemiparsis following stroke: a preliminary report, *J of Neurologic Rehab* **12** (1998), 111-8.

[15]   G. V. Smith, K. H. C. Silver, A. P. Goldberg and R. F. Macko, "Task-oriented" exercise improves hamstring strength and spastic reflexes in chronic stroke patients, *Stroke* **30** (1999), 2112-8.

[16]   E. L. Bennett, *Neural Mechanisms of Learning and Memory.* MIT Press Ltd: Cambridge, 1976.

[17]   M. Rosenzweig, Animal models for effects of brain lesions and for rehabilitation, In *Recovery of function: Theoretical considerations for brain injury.* University Park Press. Baltimore, 1980.

[18]   A-L. Ohlsson and B. B. Johansson, The environment influences functional outcome of cerebral infarction in rats, *Stroke* **26** (1995), 644-649.

[19]   M. Grabowski, J. C. Sørensen, B. Mattson, J. Zimmer and B. B. Johansson, Influence of an enriched environment and cortical grafting on functional outcome in brain infarcts in adult rats, *Experimental Neurology* **133** (1995), 1-7.

[20]   M. L. Thompson, G. W. Thickbroom, B.A. Laing, S. A. Wilson and F. L. Mastaglia, Transcranial magnetic stimulation studies of the corticomotor projection to the hand after sub-cortical stroke, *Movement Disorders* **11** (1996), 25.1.

[21]   R. Traversa, P. Cicinelli, A. B. Bassi, P. M. Rossini and G. Bernardi, Mapping of motor cortical reorganization after stroke, *Stroke* **28** (1997), 110-117.

[22]   F. D. Rose, D. A. Johnson, E. A. Attree, A. G. Leadbetter and T. K. Andrews, Virtual reality in neurological rehabilitation, *Brit J of Ther and Rehab,* **3** (1996), 223 – 228.

[23]   S. M. McDonough, J. H. Crosbie, L. Pokluda and M. D. J. McNeill, The use of virtual reality in the rehabilitation of the upper limb following hemiplegic stroke, *Proc 2nd International Workshop on Virtual Rehabilitation,* (2003), Piscataway, 98.

[24]   J. J. Kozak, P. A. Hancock, E. J. Arthur and S. T. Chrysler, Transfer of training from virtual reality. *Ergonomics,* **36** (1993), 777 – 784.

[25]   M. F. Folstein, S. E. Folstein and P. R. McHugh, Mini Mental state. A practical method for grading the cognitive state of patients for the clinician, *Journal of Psychiatric* Research **12** (1975), 189-198.

[26]   D. T. Wade, *Measurement in neurological rehabilitation,* Oxford University Press, Oxford, 1992.

[27]   M. L. Albert, A simple test of visual neglect, *Neurology* **23** (1973), 658-664.

[28]   B. G. Witmer and M. J. Singer, Measuring presence in virtual environments: A presence questionnaire. *Presenc,* **7** (1998), 225 – 240.

[29]   R. Kizony, L. Raz, N. Katz, H. Weingarden and P. L. Weiss, Using a video projected VR system for patients with spinal cord injury, *Proc 2nd International Workshop on Virtual Rehabilitation,* (2003) Piscataway, 82-88.

[30]   G. V. Borg, Psychophysical bases of perceived exertion, *Med Sci in Sport and Exe* **14** (1982), 377-381.

Personalised Health Management Systems
C.D. Nugent et al. (Eds.)
IOS Press, 2005

Monitoring of Symptoms and Interventions Associated with Multiple Sclerosis

Andrea LOWE-STRONG[1], Paul J. McCULLAGH[2]
[1]*Health and Rehabilitation Sciences Research Institute, Faculty of Life and Health Sciences*
[2]*School of Computing and Mathematics, Faculty of Engineering*
University of Ulster at Jordanstown, UK

Abstract. We have utilized the Structured Data Entry approach to build a prototype interface for the recording of personalized symptoms associated with Multiple Sclerosis (MS). The software provides both graphical input and output, to facilitate efficient data entry and monitoring. Graphical input is transformed to textual information, which is stored in a database in a hierarchical tree structure. Pain management in MS may be achieved by careful monitoring of the symptom in response to treatment. Pain location is selected on a body image and severity and other attributes represented using a graphical visual analog scale, leading to more convenient input and a less ambiguous coding than is achievable with narrative text alone. The Internet can be used to record and provide access to clinical data, assisting the citizen by providing a healthcare professional partnership approach to care. This approach could provide an objective means of monitoring symptoms and hence provide a more personalized approach to MS management.

Keywords. Multiple sclerosis, monitoring, symptoms, healthcare, personalization.

Introduction

In Mapping the Potential of eHealth [1], it is proposed that "eHealth empowers the patient, "to be more informed in their interactions with clinical professionals so that they can be aware of actions they can take in self help" and empowers the clinicians and healthcare professional "to gain access to information on patients, treatment and diagnosis from other parts of the care process, and in particular, to improve interfaces between primary and secondary care". This shift from the 'traditional' healthcare approach requires the use of information technology tools, and relies upon communications infrastructure. The Internet, and the broadband access techniques now available to many individuals (Northern Ireland has 100% broadband access), can provide the communication, but new software tools are required for recording and processing information. These tools cannot be generic for every disease process, but require input from specialists in the specific disease domains. Some domains have been quick to exploit this paradigm. For example, in diabetes, individuals can check their daily blood glucose level, which can be stored in a meter. These measures, along with insulin intake, carbohydrate intake and exercise (previously recorded in a paper diary) can be uploaded to a web site, which can assist the citizen and clinician in monitoring and controlling the disease process [2]. This provides added value and a more personalised approach to healthcare.

For multiple sclerosis (MS), the Internet based approach to citizen-professional care could also be used in monitoring control and assessing the impact of intervention. Less use has made of this approach, as many symptoms associated with MS are qualitative in nature and more difficult to computerise. However, intelligent interface design can provide an objective measure of such symptoms.

MS is a chronic inflammatory disease of the central nervous system characterised by relapses and remissions [3, 4] and is the most common cause of acquired neurological dysfunction affecting young adults [5]. It is a progressively degenerative disease characterised by inflammatory demyelination and axonal loss [6]. Plaques occur in the white matter of the central nervous system which are random and erratic in nature and are responsible for the manifestation of complex and interacting symptoms of MS that change over time [7, 8]; this leads to neurological deficits of varying degrees and intensity [9].

Many individuals present with different symptoms following each relapse [10], and consequently, it is the unpredictable nature of attacks and the resulting symptoms that contribute to the detrimental impact that this disease inflicts upon the individual [11] and their quality of life [12]. The immunomodulating agents that help to reduce and manage relapses in some individuals are only partially effective in altering the course of the disease [3, 13, 14]. Thus, treatments to alleviate symptoms remain central to the management of MS [4, 14].

Symptoms associated with MS can be classified as primary, secondary, or tertiary [15]. Primary symptoms are caused directly by the disease and can involve sensory, motor, cognitive, and behavioural functions [4]. Among the most disabling primary symptoms are spasticity, pain, incontinence [7], fatigue [16], and gait problems [17]. Secondary symptoms arise as a result of the primary symptoms and include urinary tract infections, ulcers, acquired pneumonia [4], and limited ambulation [15]. The psychosocial consequences of the disease are classified as tertiary symptoms [4, 15]. With the possibility of an individual presenting with an array of symptoms, treatment can be demoralising and frustrating for both patient and physician [10]. However, successful symptomatic treatment can improve the individual's ability to function, restore a sense of control, and enhance their quality of life [3].

Northern Ireland is recognised as having a large MS population [18]; an epidemiological study found an extremely high and increasing prevalence [19]. It is estimated that approximately 3,500 people are currently diagnosed with MS [20]. Such findings have huge implications for healthcare and societal costs (18). Disability and high morbidity are common features of MS [21]. There is (as yet) no cure and disease modifying therapies only slow the progression of the disease [22]. Therefore management of MS must be a long-term consideration.

Symptoms can be measured as a baseline and then at various stages during the course of treatment. Thus, there is obviously a role for computers to assist with the management of symptoms. With appropriate training, symptoms can be quantified (using categorical descriptors) and entered into a database by the individual themselves as opposed to the healthcare professional. This is a valid approach as self-reporting has been shown to be as reliable as clinician/researcher completion [e.g., see 23]. By using the Internet, the symptom data can be stored in a globally accessible format with appropriate security and access considerations. If data associated with these symptoms are displayed in graphical format, more effective monitoring of the symptoms and hence the condition is possible, and the impact of treatment may be verified.

Better monitoring can reduce the need for duplicate assessments and provide a more efficient citizen/clinician consultation. Potentially, this means that the clinician can provide a higher quality, cost effective consultation.

1. Structured Data Entry

Structured data entry (SDE) consists of entry of data into forms with context sensitive content, driven by a knowledge base [24]. This approach ensures data is obtained efficiently in a more complete, reliable and less ambiguous format. Data entry is best captured directly at the point of encounter. There should also be 'added value' to encourage the use of computer based patient recording by providing additional functionality which is not available by using paper-based records. For the clinician, the added value may include visual monitoring of symptoms, statistical data to aid in audits and to facilitate the process of professional appraisals and clinical governance.

Several databases specialising in MS have been compiled [25]. These include: the European Database on Multiple Sclerosis (EDMUS, *http://www.edmus.org/*), which was developed to assist practitioners with appropriate follow-up of people with MS and for dealing with research problems, such as use of tools for comparison and selection, exchanging data, and retrieving data; the North American Research Consortium on MS (NARCOMS [26]) patient registry which contains data on demographics, healthcare resources, disease status, therapies, and disability status. As the database is user driven, registrants provide a wide range of information related to their experience with MS; and, MS-COSTAR, public domain software, which provides functions for storing, retrieving, analysing, and displaying demographic, clinical, and test data for people with MS. These databases provide some standardisation on shared vocabularies for MS. For example EDMUS provides a classification of sensory functions, ranging from "normal" (quantified as 0) through to "sensation essentially lost below the head" (quantified as 6). In between scores of 1-5 are associated with the severity of limb vibration, decrease in touch, pain or position sense and proprioceptive changes in limbs. However, the recording of these symptoms is essentially as free text and classification scores.

2. User Interface

Software was developed for a standalone PC in Borland DELPHI to provide a SDE interface tailored for MS symptom entry ([27], see Figure 1). The user selects a symptom from a predefined list: *pain, weakness or numbness*. Selecting a super-imposed hot spot on a graphical image of the body then specifies the location. Attributes associated with the symptom may then be selected. Spatial direction may be selected using a compass metaphor e.g. top left icon represents north-west. A graphical Visual Analogue Scale (VAS) is used to quantify the symptom. The scale uses a line to represent the severity of pain that someone could suffer, from '*No Pain*' at one end to '*Worst Pain Ever*' at the other. The McGill Pain Questionnaire [28], an internationally recognized and validated measure of recording pain, is the basis for the description of the symptoms. Information is provided for *type, frequency and duration*. Type is distinguished using one of the following nineteen categories: *annoying, boring, burning, cool, crushing, cutting, dull, flashing, frightful, itchy, nagging, numb, piercing, pounding, sickening, splitting, tiring, tugging, vicious*. Frequency may be set as follows: *per minute, per hour, per day, per night, per week, per month*. Duration may be set as follows: *seconds, minutes, hours, days, weeks, months, continuous*. Where additional free text is required to accompany the pre-defined categories in the record, checking the '*additional information box*' provides a pop up text entry window.

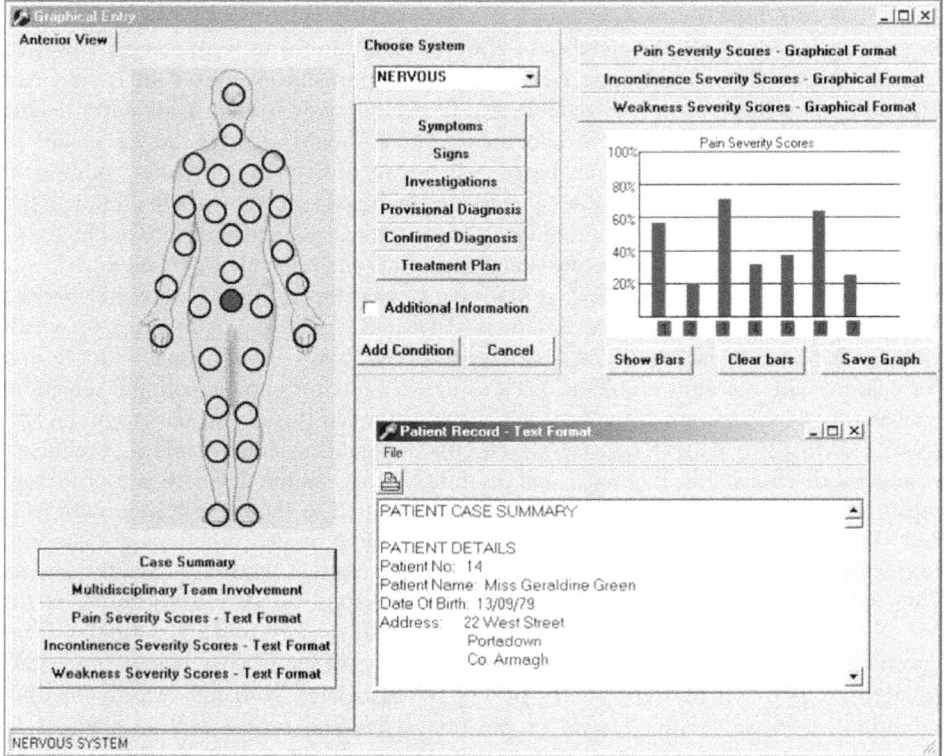

Figure 1. Data Input and Output with symptom trends and summary.

Other symptoms such as weakness and numbness may be specified in a similar fashion. Figure 1 also shows how a symptom can be tracked over time, and that a textual output can be printed.

3. Internet Based Monitoring

The SDE prototype described in section 3 was implemented for standalone PC. This permitted the interface to be tested and the usefulness of the approach to be assessed. However, this software solution does not fit well with the intended end user, i.e. the individual at home. The Internet and the progress made with ubiquitous access over broadband connections provide many advantages:

- It permits a 'thin client' solution, where the citizen can enter details and access results using a conventional browser, but is not responsible for the upkeep of the central database.
- It permits a communication platform for the user and the healthcare professional. Indeed, in this scenario, the user can control the data providing access to trusted healthcare professionals. The diabetes monitoring domain has led the way with this care model.
- It provides potential for interoperability of the self monitored symptoms with the electronic patient record, provided that appropriate standards are used in its implementations. These include standard security safeguards.
- It provides the possibility to support research, using data processing to study the relationship between interventions and disease control.

An Internet-base solution requires a re-engineering of the software. An initial implementation used Internet Information Services, Active Server Pages (ASP.NET and Web Matrix development environment) and Microsoft SQL Server to demonstrate that this solution was feasible for a desktop client. However, we propose a more flexible open architecture, with a thin client, possibly a personal digital assistant (PDA) for data collection and display. Data Interchange and interoperability will be facilitated by an extensible markup language (XML). A three-tier architecture comprising:

- presentation server: Apache, the predominant cross platform server.
- application server: PHP, a scripting language embedded in hypertext markup language and Simple Object Access Protocol, an XML based protocol to let applications exchange information over the hypertext transfer protocol.
- database server: MySQL provides an open, cross platform and scalable solution.

The end user device can be partially connected, permitting local data capture and subsequent upload. For a mobile device such as a PDA, the graphical SDE is particularly appropriate given the usability restrictions associated with the smaller screen size, and more difficult textual input. Where the individual is unable to use the input device due to the progression of the illness, symptoms can be entered by a caregiver or healthcare professional, e.g. health visitor or clinician.

4. Conclusions

The graphical SDE described in this paper could contribute to efficient data entry and retrieval in the MS domain to facilitate citizen/clinician communication. The prototype interface is straightforward and may be suitable for self-monitoring of symptoms, by individuals with MS. This approach is appropriate to an Internet based implementation, and we propose a scalable cross platform solution, which will support open standards and interoperability. Such an implementation could assist with personalized decision support, by making it easier for the citizen and healthcare professional to extract relevant information.

References

[1] Wilson P. Mapping the potential of eHealth: Empowering the citizen through eHealth tools and services. eHealth Conference, Cork, 5-6 May 2004. European Institute of Public Administration

[2]   Accu-Chek,http://www.accu-chek.com/products/data_compass.jsp
[3]   Lisak D. Overview of symptomatic management of multiple sclerosis. *J Neurosci Nurs* 2001; 33(5): 224-30
[4]   Jonsson A, Ravnborg MH. Rehabilitation in multiple sclerosis. *Crit Rev Phys Rehab Medicine* 1998; 10(1): 75-100
[5]   Barcellos LF, Thomson G. Genetic Analysis of Multiple Sclerosis in Europeans. *J Neuroimmunol* 2003; 143 (1-2): 1-6
[6]   Amor S, Layward L, Van Noort JM. Multiple Sclerosis: Modeling The Future. The Multiple Sclerosis Society of Great Britain and Northern Ireland Conference: Frontiers in Science and Patient Care Disease Management. *Mol Med Today* 1998; 4(8): 328-30
[7]   KoKo C. Effectiveness of rehabilitation for multiple sclerosis. *Clin Rehab* 1999; 13(1): 33-41
[8]   Smith KJ, McDonald WI. The pathophysiology of multiple sclerosis: the mechanisms underlying the production of symptoms and the natural history of the disease. *Philos Trans R Soc Lond B Biol Sci 1999; 354: 1649-73*
[9]   Jonsson A, Ravnborg MH. Rehabilitation in Multiple Sclerosis. *Critical Reviews in Physical and Rehabilitation Medicine* 1998; 10(1): 75-100
[10].   Whitney DK. Early diagnosis and intervention in multiple sclerosis. *Int J MS care* 2001; 3(3): 1-9
[11]   Rao SM, Huber SJ, Bornstein RA. Emotional changes with Multiple Sclerosis and Parkinson's disease. *J Consult Clin Psychol* 1992; 60:369-78
[12]   Brassat D, Clanet M. Treatment of symptoms and relapses of multiple sclerosis. *Rev Prat (French).* 1999; 49 (17): 187-71
[13]   Miltenburger C, Kobelt G. Quality of life and cost of multiple sclerosis. Clinical Neurol Neurosurg 2002; 104: 27-25
[14]   Leary SM, Thompson AJ Current management of multiple sclerosis. *Int J Clin Pract* 2000; 54(3): 16-19
[15]   Bever, CT. Multiple Sclerosis: symptomatic treatment. *Current Treat Options Neurol* 1999; 1:221-37
[16]   Thompson AJ. Symptomatic management and rehabilitation in multiple sclerosis. *J Neurol Neurosurg Psych* 2001; 71 (2): 22-27
[17]   Morris ME, Cantwell C, Vowels L, Dodd K. Changes in gait and fatigue from morning to afternoon in people with multiple sclerosis. *J Neurol Neurosurg Psych* 2002; 72: 361-5
[18]   McDonnell GV, Hawkins SA. Multiple Sclerosis in Northern Ireland: a historical and global perspective. *Ulster Med J* 2000; 69(2): 97-105
[19]   McDonnell GV, Hawkins SA (1998). An epidemiologic study of multiple sclerosis in Northern Ireland. *Neurol* 1998; 50: 423-28
[20]   MS Society, Northern Ireland http://www.mssocietyni.co.uk Accessed 8th March 2005
[21]   Davis WM. Multiple Sclerosis: Continuing Mysteries and Current Management. *Drug Topics* 2000; 144 (12): 93-102
[22]   Polman CH, Uitdehaag BM. Drug Treatment of Multiple Sclerosis. *Brit Med J* 2000; 321 (7259): 490–494
[23]   Groom MJ, Lincoln NB, Francis VM, Stephan TF. Assessing mood in patients with multiple sclerosis. *Clin Rehabil* 2003; 17(8): 847-857
[24]   van Ginneken AM, Moorman, PW and Brecht AA. The patient record. In: van Bemmel, JH, Musen, MA, eds, *Handbook of Medical Informatics*, Springer, 1997; pp. 99-115
[25]   Reports From the 2000 Annual Meetings of Rehabilitation in Multiple Sclerosis and the Consortium of Multiple Sclerosis Centers. The current state of MS Databases, *International Journal of MS Care* (Supplement), 2000: 2(3). http://www.mscare.com
[26]   Vollmer TL, Ni W, Stanton S, Hadjimichael O. The NARCOMS patient registry: A resource for investigators. *International Journal of MS Care* 1999: 1: pp.12-15. http://www.mscare.com
[27]   McCullagh PJ, McGuigan J, Fegan M, Lowe-Strong A. Structured Data Entry using Graphical Input: Recording Symptoms for Multiple Sclerosis. *Studies in Health Technology and Informatics* 95: 673-678, eds R Baud et al, 2003
[28]   Melzack R. The McGill Pain Questionnaire: major properties and scoring methods. *Pain* 1: 1975: pp. 277-99

Personalised Health Management Systems
C.D. Nugent et al. (Eds.)
IOS Press, 2005

Intelligent Analysis of EMG Data for Improving Lifestyle

Mark DONNELLY, Richard DAVIES, Chris NUGENT
School of Computing and Mathematics, Faculty of Engineering
University of Ulster at Jordanstown, Northern Ireland

Abstract. In the tragic situation when a person loses his or her hand, they are usually faced with only one option if they wish to regain a good level of mobility; learn to control an artificial hand. It has been suggested that our brain stores a "body map" of the different parts in our body. Thus, if a person loses a hand, their "body map" remains intact and produces phantom sensations that permit the person to feel like they still have their hand. Some discomfort is felt during these sensations; nevertheless, there is a positive side to them as they enable patients to control prosthetic replacements. Sensations experienced can be measured using a method known as Electromyography (EMG) and can be acquired and processed to control an artificial hand. This research involved the acquisition, analysis and classification of EMG signals through construction of a recording device and the development of classification models based on heuristic approaches and Artificial Intelligence classifiers based on Neural Networks to control artificial hands.

Keywords. Electromyography, Artificial Hand, Signal Processing, Neural Networks.

Introduction

The human hand is a vital part of the human anatomy and has a wide range of practical uses. It is controlled by our central nervous system with the lower levels of our brain co-coordinating the fingers and joints. Most human activities revolve around the use of our hands to help complete everyday tasks. Without the use of our hands even the simplest tasks can become time consuming and in some cases impossible to complete. Due to current miniaturisation in consumer products, tasks are becoming more problematic for amputees as new devices become smaller thus assisting to alienate amputees from the main stream hence reducing their quality of life.

Conventional artificial hands fall into two categories: Functional and Cosmetic. For Functional, the prosthetic is a mechanical device such as a hook that provides the basic forms of grip, precision and power [1]. In Cosmetic the hand has a life-like appearance but is fixed in a precision grip so it is non-functional or compliant. Conventional prosthetic hand devices only offer simple functions like grasping motions [1]. They use the electrical signals emanated from the forearm in a limited way. For example, two muscles could be used to instruct an artificial hand, one used to open the hand and one used to close it.

In interacting with small objects our fingers play a major role and are fundamental in the completion of such dexterous tasks. Consequently, it seems intuitive to suggest that future artificial hand devices should address the ability to control finger movements as opposed to grasping like motions.

The aims of this research were two fold. Firstly, to develop a device capable of recording electrical signals from the anterior region of a forearm and secondly, based on these recorded signals, to develop a set of classifiers that could discriminate between different individual finger movements. The expected benefits will offer the ability to control the finger movements of a prosthetic device thus permitting amputees to perform more dexterous tasks.

1. EMG data collection

In order to develop a set of classifiers to discriminate between finger movements a data set was obtained using a custom built EMG recording device. Surface EMG is an ideal control signal to obtain as it provides plentiful information in a non-invasive manner. The recordings were taken from the anterior region of a forearm using two surface mounted gel electrodes.

The electrodes were coupled to a pre-amplifier operating in bi-polar mode producing a single EMG channel thus minimising any common noise. The usable energy in an EMG signal ranges from 0 to 500 Hertz (Hz), with most of the EMG energy being contained within the 50 to 150 Hz range [2]. Nevertheless, the frequency components between 0 and 20 Hz are known to be unstable due to the quasi-random nature in the firing rate of the motor units [2]. To simplify matters a band pass filter was implemented to remove the random signals from 0 to 20 Hz and any other unwanted energy over 500 Hz.

To utilise the full dynamic range of the Analogue to Digital Converter the signal was prepared by means of a scaling and offset module before final digitisation. Finger flexion and extension movements were repeated twelve times per finger yielding a total of forty eight recordings which formed the basis of the data set. Under control of a Reduced Instruction Set Computer the EMG signal was digitally transmitted to a host PC for further analysis. An overview of the EMG acquisition and processing is detailed in Figure 1.

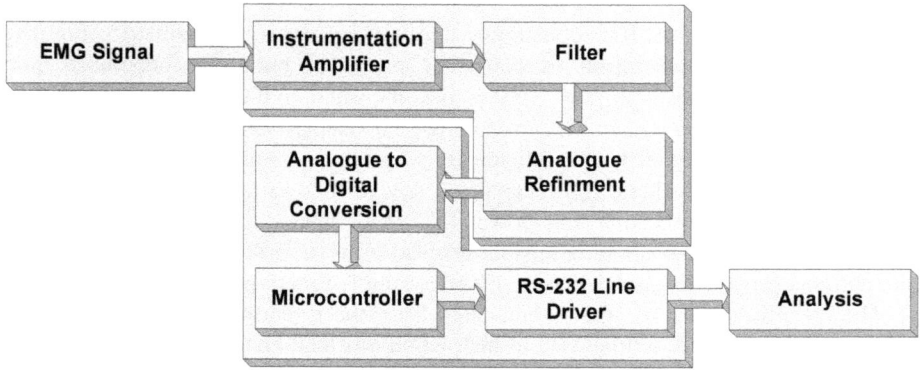

Figure 1. Overview of hardware employed for EMG signal acquisition and pre-processing.

2. EMG Classification

The aim of the second part of the research was to engineer a high quality, functional interface to effectively analyse and classify the EMG signals for the theoretical control of an artificial hand. Figure 2 provides a high level design of the components developed. These may be summarised as follows:

- Input to the system is read from a memory store containing EMG signals.
- Processing is carried out using an analysis program which provides access to a number of algorithms developed to predict finger movements.
- Two separate outputs are provided by the system.
  - o An analysis program provides graphs and tabular data, which shown the efficiency and accuracy of the processing (Figure 3).
  - o A separate program provides output through a form of animation that emulates an artificial hand and individual finger movements (Figure 4).

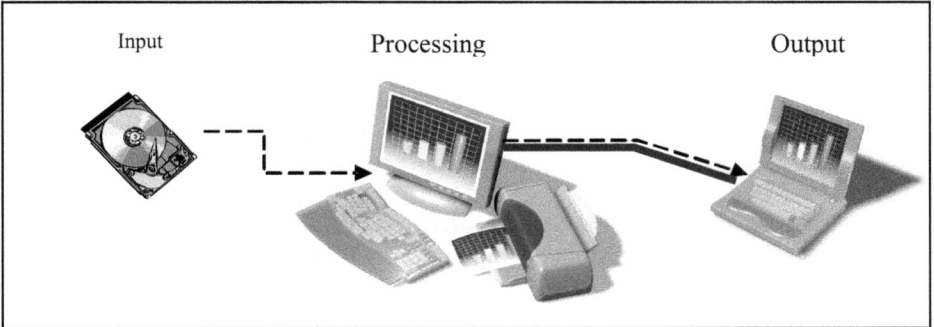

Figure 2. High level design of developed system.

For the purposes of evaluation two interfaces were developed, one to permit management and classification of the EMG signals and one to demonstrate the classification result through a 3D animation of a finger movement. The interfaces developed and used are shown in Figures 3 and 4.

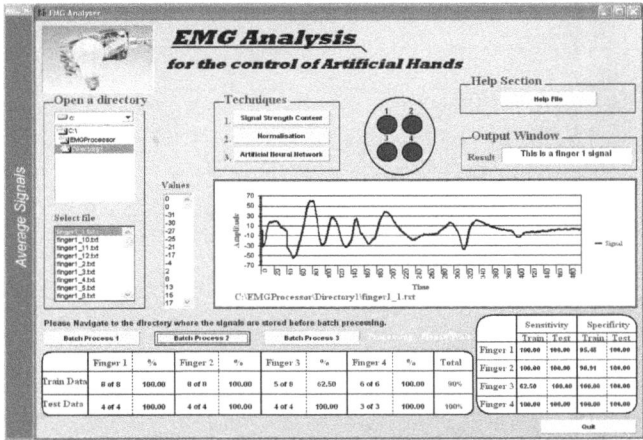

Figure 3. Interface developed for the management and processing of EMG signals.

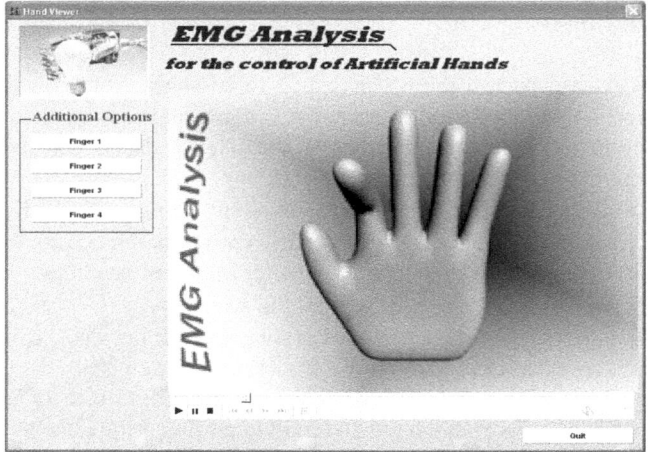

Figure 4. Interface to display results of EMG signal analysis.

In total, three algorithms were developed to classify the EMG signals into one of the four possible finger movements recorded. The first algorithm developed adopted a novel approach to analyse the signals while the second algorithm adopted a conventional heuristic approach, examining the characteristics of the different EMG signals in order to establish similarities. The final algorithm focused on the development of a Neural Network (NN). N-fold cross validation was used to verify that the results obtained from testing were not coincidence but a rational statement regarding the performance of the classifiers developed. What follows is a brief description of each classifier developed and the results obtained.

2.1. Algorithm 1 - Normalisation

This algorithm, based largely around the principles of Normalisation, was used as the benchmark from which the other classifier's performance was compared. Figure 5 highlights an extract of code describing its fundamental operation.

```
//Normalises the EMG files to look for the least differences.
int analyse2 (char File_name[])              //File name is passed in
{
    //The missing code loops 4 times to read in 4 files, containing average values, storing them in separate
    //arrays; data_array[0][xx] contains 1st average file etc. Similarly the test file values are stored in compare[xx].

        pos = 9999;                                  //Set large value to inialise variable
        for (i = 0; i < 4; i++){                     //Outer Loop
            sumof = 0;                               //Initialise variable
            for (int j = 0; j < DATA_SIZE; j++){     //Inner Loop
                a = data_array[i][j];                //Compare the file read in with each of the
                b = compare[j];                      // average files read in initially
                if (a < 0)                           //If either value is less than zero then convert
                    a = sqrt(a * a);  // it into positive value
                if (b < 0)
                    b = sqrt(b * b);
                if (b > a)                           //Ensure that the lesser value is subtracted
                    sumof += b - a; // form the higher value in order to find the difference.
                else
                    sumof += a - b;                  //End Inner Loop
            if (sumof < pos){                        //Used to keep track of the file with the least difference
                pos = sumof;
                finger = i + 1;                      //As array starts at zero, one must be added to finger.
            }
        }                                            //End Outer Loop
        return (finger);                             //Return finger
}                                                    //End finger.
```

Figure 5. Excerpt of code presenting the operation of Algorithm 1.

This was a novel approach based on the comparison of unknown signals with representative temporal templates from each of the four possible finger movements. The representative templates were compared, in turn, with the unknown signal presented and a difference measure calculated. The template offering the lowest measure of difference with the unknown signal was selected as the most likely finger movement. Following 3-fold cross validation, accuracy levels of 66.7% were attained.

2.2. Algorithm 2 - Signal strength content

A heuristic approach to classification was employed to examine the signal strength content of the training data to assess certain predefined characteristics. The algorithm concentrated on the following aspects of the signal. A signal, when displayed as a temporal recording, can be divided into three sections vertically and three sections horizontally as illustrated in Figure 6. Any values lying above the upper horizontal line were seen as high values, those between the lines as middle values and those below the lower horizontal line as low values. Similarly, only those values that fell before the left vertical line were considered as high values, those in the middle as middle values and those values following the right vertical line as low values.

This was the starting point from which the algorithm evolved. The training signals were studied to examine the characteristics they demonstrated and to determine the similarities between those signals representing the same finger movement. If the majority of signals representing a particular movement lay within a particular region of the graph then this was viewed as a characteristic of a specific finger movement.

Characteristics considered worthy were identified following the analysis described above. Applying a 3-fold cross validation procedure this algorithm produced an impressive accuracy of 93.6%.

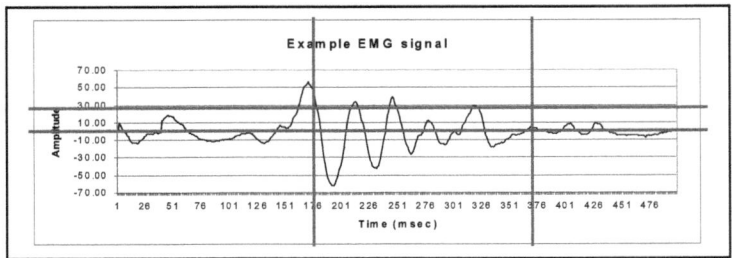

Figure 6. Screen representation of segmentation of regions of interest in training signals.

2.3. Algorithm 3 - Neural Network

The third classifier developed to classify the EMG signals was a NN. NNs have established themselves as powerful tools, especially within the realms of classification and have been used to classify many complex and large-scale problems. In general terms, they can be considered as a vast collection of densely interconnected computational elements working in parallel to solve a particular problem [3]. Their computing power is derived not only through their parallel structure but also through their ability to learn and therefore generalise, where generalisation can be considered to be the ability to produce a correct output from unseen inputs not encountered during training.

A 2 layer multi-layered perceptron with 7 nodes in the hidden layer was trained. Following initial testing accuracy levels of 100% were achieved, however, when 3-fold cross validation was applied this figure was reduced resulting in an overall classification accuracy of 67.5%. This result does not reflect the true potential of such an approach. We believe that the NN was over trained on the training set hence causing an 'over-fitting' phenomenon. Retraining employing a feature extraction algorithm permitted the NN to afford better generalisation, however, the results of this have not as yet been collated and so are not presented in this evaluation.

3. Conclusion

Upon examining the aims and objectives stated at the outset of the research it is felt that overall these have been achieved. Hardware and software has been engineered to effectively capture, analyse, evaluate and classify EMG signals for the control of an artificial hand. This has been achieved through background research to compare and evaluate different methods of signal capture and by developing software to implement the analysis methods chosen. Combining the performance from all three techniques resulted in an overall average of 76% of the EMG signals being correctly classified. By increasing the size of the data set, i.e. number of training finger movements, it is anticipated that the performance and stability of the algorithms will be further improved.

This work has shown that careful evaluation of EMG signals have the potential to be used to control finger movements in artificial hands. Although the algorithms require a form of 'learning' prior to being able to classify EMG signals into one of four possible finger movements this can be seen as an advantage. Such an approach would require the end user to train the device, hence, each system would be specifically 'personalised' to the individual characteristics of the EMG signal for different finger movements for each user.

References

[1]   P. J. Kyberd, M. Evans, S. Te Winkel, "An intelligent Anthropomorphic Hand, with Automatic Grasp," *Robotica*, 16, pp. 531-536, 1998.
[2]   C.J. De Luca, "The use of surface electromyography in biomechanics," *Journal of Applied Biomechanics*, vol. 13, 2, pp. 135-163, 1997.
[3]   R. Lippmann, "An introduction to computing with neural nets," *IEEE ASSP*, vol. 4, 2, pp. 4-22, 1987.

Personalised Health Management Systems
C.D. Nugent et al. (Eds.)
IOS Press, 2005

235

Author Index

www.ingramcontent.com/pod-product-compliance
Ingram Content Group UK Ltd.
Pitfield, Milton Keynes, MK11 3LW, UK
UKHW050242300526
471096UK00013B/9